Psychological Insights for Understanding COVID-19 and Health

With specially commissioned introductions from international experts, the *Psychological Insights for Understanding COVID-19* series draws together previously published chapters on key themes in psychological science that engage with people's unprecedented experience of the pandemic.

In this volume on health, Dominika Kwasnicka and Robbert Sanderman introduce chapters that explore the crucial topics of health behaviour change, wellbeing, stress, and coping. They highlight the key role digital health technologies can play in how we manage health conditions, and how we facilitate change to help individuals manage stressful situations such as physical isolation, job loss, and financial strain during the COVID-19 pandemic. The volume also offers an important overview of environmental and policy-based approaches to health behaviour change and addresses the highly relevant issues of identity and trust and how they shape the health of individuals, communities, and society.

Highlighting theory and research on these key topics germane to the global pandemic, the *Psychological Insights for Understanding COVID-19* series offers thought-provoking reading for professionals, students, academics, and policymakers concerned with psychological consequences of COVID-19 for individuals, families, and society.

Dr Dominika Kwasnicka is Research Fellow at the NHMRC Centre of Research Excellence in Digital Technology to Transform Chronic Disease Outcomes, University of Melbourne, Australia, and SWPS University of Social Sciences and Humanities, Poland. She is a behavioural scientist with diverse interests in health psychology, digital health, and research methods focusing on individuals.

Prof Dr Robbert Sanderman is Professor in Health Psychology at both the University of Groningen and at the University of Twente, The Netherlands. His research focuses on psychological and social adaptation to chronic life-threatening illness and on the use of psychological interventions, including eHealth tools.

The editors lead – together with others – the Open Digital Health initiative (www.opendigitalhealth.org) that promotes reusing open digital health solutions across contexts and settings.

Psychological Insights for Understanding COVID-19

The *Psychological Insights for Understanding COVID-19* series aims to highlight important themes in psychological science that engage with people's unprecedented experience of the COVID-19 pandemic. These short, accessible volumes draw together chapters as they originally appeared before COVID-19 descended on the world but demonstrate how researchers and professionals in psychological science had developed theory and research on key topics germane to the global pandemic. Each volume includes a specially commissioned, expert introduction that contextualises the chapters in relation to the crisis, reflects on the relevance of psychological research during this significant global event, and proposes future research and vital interventions that elucidate understanding and coping with COVID-19. With individual volumes exploring society, health, family, work and media, the *Psychological Insights for Understanding COVID-19* series offers thought-provoking reading for professionals, students, academics and policy makers concerned with psychological consequences of the pandemic for individuals, families and society.

Titles in the series:

Psychological Insights for Understanding COVID-19 and Families, Parents, and Children
Edited by Marc H. Bornstein

Psychological Insights for Understanding COVID-19 and Media and Technology
Edited by Ciarán Mc Mahon

Psychological Insights for Understanding COVID-19 and Society
Edited by S. Alexander Haslam

Psychological Insights for Understanding COVID-19 and Work
Edited by Cary L. Cooper

Psychological Insights for Understanding COVID-19 and Health
Edited by Dominika Kwasnicka and Robbert Sanderman

For more information about this series, please visit: https://www.routledge.com/Psychological-Insights-for-Understanding-COVID-19/book-series/COVID

Psychological Insights for Understanding COVID-19 and Health

Edited by Dominika Kwasnicka
and Robbert Sanderman

Routledge
Taylor & Francis Group
LONDON AND NEW YORK

First published 2021
by Routledge
2 Park Square, Milton Park, Abingdon, Oxon OX14 4RN

and by Routledge
52 Vanderbilt Avenue, New York, NY 10017

Routledge is an imprint of the Taylor & Francis Group, an informa business

British Library Cataloguing-in-Publication Data
A catalogue record for this book is available from the British Library

Library of Congress Cataloging-in-Publication Data
A catalog record for this book has been requested

ISBN: 978-0-367-69238-4 (hbk)
ISBN: 978-0-367-68965-0 (pbk)
ISBN: 978-1-003-14109-9 (ebk)

Typeset in Times New Roman
by Apex CoVantage, LLC

Selected chapters are taken from the following original Routledge publications

Health Psychology: An Interdisciplinary Approach
Deborah Fish Ragin
ISBN: 978-1-138-20130-9 (hbk) ISBN: 978-13-155-1229-7 (ebk)

The Psychology of Wellbeing
Gary W. Wood
ISBN: 978-0-367-89809-0 (hbk) ISBN: 978-0-367-89808-3 (pbk)
ISBN: 978-1-003-02125-4 (ebk)

eHealth Research, Theory and Development: A Multidisciplinary Approach
Edited by Lisette van Gemert-Pijnen, Saskia M. Kelders, Hanneke Kip, and Robbert Sanderman
ISBN: 978-1-138-23042-2 (hbk) ISBN: 978-1-138-23043-9 (pbk)
ISBN: 978-1-315-38590-7 (ebk)

Digital Health: Critical and Cross-Disciplinary Perspectives
Deborah Lupton
ISBN: 978-1-138-12344-1 (hbk) ISBN: 978-1-138-12345-8 (pbk)
ISBN: 978-1-315-64883-5 (ebk)

Health Behavior Change: Theories, Methods and Interventions
Andrew Prestwich, Jared B. Kenworthy, Mark Conner
ISBN: 978-1-138-69481-1 (hbk) ISBN: 978-1-138-69482-8 (pbk)
ISBN: 978-1-315-52721-5 (ebk)

Motivation for Sustaining Health Behavior Change: The Self-as-Doer Identity
Amanda M. Brouwer
ISBN: 978-1-138-03635-2 (hbk) ISBN: 978-0-367-26633-2 (pbk)
ISBN: 978-1-315-17865-3 (ebk)

The Psychology of Trust
Ken J. Rotenberg
ISBN: 978-1-138-67848-4 (hbk) ISBN: 978-1-138-67849-1 (pbk)
ISBN: 978-1-315-55891-2 (ebk)

Contents

Contributors

Amanda M. Brouwer, Associate Professor, Psychology Department, Winona State University, USA.

Mark Conner, Professor, School of Psychology, University of Leeds, UK.

Deborah Fish Ragin, Professor Emeritus, Montclair State University, USA.

Matthew Howard, Director of Artificial Intelligence at Deloitte, UK.

Saskia M. Kelders, Associate Professor, Department of Psychology, Health and Technology, University of Twente, Enschede, the Netherlands.

Jared B. Kenworthy, Associate Professor, Department of Psychology, University of Texas Arlington, USA.

Hanneke Kip, Lecturer, Department of Psychology, Health and Technology, University of Twente, Enschede, the Netherlands.

Dominika Kwasnicka, Research Fellow, NHMRC Centre of Research Excellence in Digital Technology to Transform Chronic Disease Outcomes, University of Melbourne, Australia, and SWPS University of Social Sciences and Humanities, Poland.

Deborah Lupton, SHARP Professor in the Centre for Social Research in Health and the Social Policy Research Centre, University of New South Wales, Australia.

Andrew Prestwich, Senior Lecturer, School of Psychology, University of Leeds, UK.

Ken J. Rotenberg, School of Psychology, Keele University, UK.

Robbert Sanderman, Professor, Department of Health Psychology, University Medical Center Groningen, University of Groningen, Groningen, The Netherlands and Department of Psychology, Health and Technology, University of Twente, Enschede, The Netherlands.

Lisette van Gemert-Pijnen, Professor of Persuasive Health Technology, Department of Psychology, Health and Technology, University of Twente, Enschede, the Netherlands.

Gary W. Wood, chartered psychologist, solution-focused life coach, advice columnist, and broadcaster.

Introduction

Dominika Kwasnicka and Robbert Sanderman

Introduction

Psychological Perspectives on COVID-19 and Health aims to highlight some of the most topical themes with which psychological science will need to engage following COVID-19. The aim of this chapter is to introduce each of the chapters included in this book, describe how they are relevant to emerging norms, and contextualise the chapters in relation to the crisis, reflecting on the relevance of psychological research during this significant global event. This volume provides a thought-provoking read for professionals, students, academics, and policy makers concerned with psychological consequences of the current pandemic for individuals, families, and society. The included chapters have three overarching themes, they: (1) address health behaviour change and wellbeing; (2) explore issues of stress and coping; and (3) outline how digital health technologies can be used to facilitate health behaviour change to help individuals cope with stressful situations such as physical isolation, job loss, and financial strain during the COVID-19 pandemic.

The current pandemic is unprecedented in terms of the global spread and its widespread impact on individuals, communities, and society as a whole (Sachs et al., 2020). The impact of COVID-19 is particularly prominent in terms of its burden on the healthcare system and economy (Nicola et al., 2020). The pandemic provides a unique opportunity to rethink how we interact with each other, how we work, and how our behaviour impacts the environment (Anderson et al., 2020; Howarth et al., 2020). Behaviour change during COVID-19 is particularly relevant in terms of forming new habitual behaviours such as frequent handwashing, physical distancing, and wearing face masks (Van Bavel et al., 2020). Governments around the world implement policies that aim to slow down and stop the spread of the virus (Jee, 2020). We are being introduced to new safety measures encouraging us to stay at home, to physically socialise less, to minimise our movement, and to contact trace (Hellewell et al., 2020). These changes often come at the expense of us becoming more stressed, feeling anxious, and often struggling to cope (Polizzi et al., 2020). Children require home schooling, and parents have to balance working from home and parenting; online work presents new complexities and challenges; and relationships with people living with us are often at strain. The psychology research presented in this volume provides some suggestions for how to best deal with these new circumstances.

Digital technologies are applied around the world to facilitate implementation of new behaviours. We are encouraged to socialise and interact with our work colleagues online, and to minimise our travel for work and leisure. Healthcare was forced to move almost instantly to telehealth and online delivery, to minimise the risk of virus exposure among the most vulnerable individuals (Wosik et al., 2020). The measures are in place to shield and protect the most vulnerable, for instance, individuals who are immunocompromised, elderly, and people with chronic conditions such as chronic obstructive pulmonary disease and asthma (McKee & Stuckler, 2020). Coordinated efforts aim to motivate and encourage people to work collaboratively to slow the spread of the virus and to protect the most vulnerable. The common slogan is *'We are in this together'* meaning if we work together, we can jointly stop the spread of COVID-19. This is the beginning of a new world as we know it, and psychology plays a great role in terms of promoting health behaviour change and helping people to cope with new challenges faced during a pandemic. Digital health solutions play a significant role in how we manage health conditions, interact with healthcare professionals, and access health information and the most suitable healthcare.

This volume brings together relevant chapters that will encourage the reader to see the current world through the prism of psychological theory, to improve emotional health and wellbeing, and to cope better with COVID-19-related stress. The readers' attention will be drawn to new opportunities of technology to promote health and wellbeing and to learn about the lived experience of using digital health. This volume will also give an overview of environmental and policy-based approaches to health behaviour change. Even though the chapter on this topic, like also most of the other chapters, was written prior to the pandemic, the issue of environmental and contextual influences on behaviour change is particularly relevant now, when new rules and laws are being introduced to protect health. Around the world, people respond differently to newly emerging norms, and that often impacts the effectiveness of new policies to decrease virus spread. We witnessed very clear messaging and coordinated response in New Zealand and relatively unclear messaging and resistance movements in the United States, and the two countries success in stopping the virus spread has been visibly different. The final chapters of this volume address the highly relevant issues of identity, trust, and health, and will demonstrate how these constructs are interconnected and how they shape the health of individuals, communities, and society.

Chapters' overview

In the opening chapter 'Emotional health and wellbeing', Deborah Fish Ragin defines and compares four major models of health and wellbeing; that is, the biomedical, biopsychosocial, wellness, and ecological models, all developed and tested in the 20th century, largely in Western cultures representing a modern view of health. The biomedical model places biology at the core of the definition of health, i.e., health is defined as absence of disease (e.g., being COVID-19 free); biopsychosocial model expands on the definition by including psychological, social, and emotional wellbeing (e.g., coping well with the pandemic psychologically, socially and emotionally); the wellness model adds two new dimensions: quality of life and spirituality. The ecological model adds contextual dimensions: physical and psychological environments, health systems, and health policy. The ecological model seems the most suitable to define health in times of the pandemic when our health and wellbeing is not only defined by absence of disease (being COVID-19 free), but more importantly by maintaining social connections (keeping physical distance) and living in a society where people are safe and protected. In line with the ecological model, people need to work jointly to minimise disease spread, to ensure that the healthcare system can cope with dramatically increasing demand on services, and that health policy protects all citizens.

In this chapter Deborah Fish Ragin also defines and criticises positive psychology, giving three examples of studies looking at the influence of positive affect on health. Positive psychology emphasises that positive emotions, experiences, and personal characteristics contribute to positive, healthy outcomes. Positive psychology builds on the wellness model of health and involves a systematic study of the factors that enhance and maintain an individual's state of wellbeing. According to studies presented in this chapter, personal traits such as subjective wellbeing, optimism, happiness, self-determination, and positive emotional states contribute to positive psychology and wellbeing. This is worth keeping in mind when observing our own response to new COVID-19 realities. Similarly, recent study suggests that optimists, those with a high level of general trust, showed lower levels of fear and higher levels of preventive behaviours in relation to COVID-19; pessimists on the other hand, show higher level of fear (Jovančević & Milićević, 2020). With other studies showing that on the contrary, optimistically biased respondents perceived their risk of COVID-19 to be low and they were less likely to undertake protective behaviours (Park et al., 2020). With no consensus on the topic of optimism and engaging in COVID-19 protective behaviours, we encourage the reader to remain optimistic about the future, while adopting protective behaviours and following national guidelines.

Finally, in this chapter Deborah Fish Ragin describes three major types of traditional medicine; that is, Chinese, folk medicines (e.g., *curanderismo* and *sangoma*), and Native American healing practices, and looks into differences between traditional and modern medicine. Most traditional medicines share core principles including a connection among the individual, Earth, and energy force, a balance of these connected elements and the use of herbal remedies or other practices such as ritual chants and acupuncture. The World Health Organization made it clear that traditional medicine is not an effective treatment for COVID-19; despite this, there have been reports of the use of traditional medicine as a treatment for patients with COVID-19 (Xiao & Torok, 2020). Understanding different models of health and wellbeing, and learning about positive psychology can help the reader interpret the impact of COVID-19 on individuals and healthcare systems. Learning about different approaches to medicine, including traditional medicine, highlights different perspectives on COVID-19 treatment, the disease that has already spread through 213 countries and territories around the world and is still on the rise globally.

The next chapter by Gary W. Wood could not be more topical during the pandemic, as it addresses stress and coping. The recent events have been particularly stressful, especially for people who are directly affected by COVID-19; that is, people who have been infected, their social networks, and healthcare workers who are dealing with highly infectious virus, especially those who test and treat infected people (Wang et al., 2020). The healthcare system in many countries is overwhelmed by the pandemic and healthcare professionals often struggle to cope with limited resources, for example lack of hospital beds, ventilators, and protective equipment (Grasselli et al., 2020). Patients can be extremely stressed and anxious, and need to be physically isolated to protect their relatives. COVID-19 has redefined the way we live, shop, and travel. It has affected most of us as we live under COVID-19 restrictions, and, even if not directly affected by the disease, we can experience stress, anxiety, and boredom.

In Chapter 2 Gary W. Wood looks at normality, adjustment, and positive mental health and wellbeing, exploring the tension between survival and safety, and personal growth. He suggests that the way we define stress determines how we cope with stressors. Particularly relevant to the COVID-19 world is the section describing emotion-focused coping, which involves trying to reduce negative emotional responses associated with stress, such as sadness, fear, or frustration. The examples of emotion-focused coping are distraction (watching TV), exercising, journaling, praying, engaging in mindfulness, breathing techniques, or talking to others (friends, psychologists). All suggested techniques of dealing with stress are particularly relevant solutions for people living under lockdown restrictions. Control-focused strategies that are also relevant to dealing with COVID-19-related stress aim to address the source of the issue causing stress, and often involve problem solving, improving time-management, learning, or getting support. Strategies may also include getting more information to re-evaluate the problem, for instance, 'I am relatively safe if I follow the guidelines such as staying at home, minimising physical contact, wearing mask'. This chapter also covers the role of cognitive appraisal and presents theories from psychology and coaching with practical suggestions for how to cope. These include the hassles and uplifts theory, psychological hardiness, and learning skills. This knowledge can be applied when developing behavioural interventions. The chapter concludes with a review of the research on mindfulness and outcomes in psychotherapy and counselling. It offers advice on getting support and invites the reader to reflect on the 'new normal'.

The third chapter by Saskia M. Kelders and Matthew Howard is titled 'Opportunities of technology to promote health and well-being'; this chapter relates to the chapters on health behaviour change and stress and coping. When and how we can use technology to influence behaviour are explained. For example, preventing the spread of the virus – as in the case of the use of track-and-trace applications (Whitelaw et al., 2020). The authors illustrate how technology could support individuals to cope with stress, and the effects of COVID-19 in patients and others (e.g., family, healthcare workers). Also, the authors give a brief overview of the design process, which aligns with the next chapter by Lupton, addressing stakeholders' involvement (van Gemert-Pijnen et al., 2018). Kelders and Howard describe the fast pace of innovation and issues that simultaneously slow down the implementation of technology. The rapid innovation ('digital revolution') is no doubt beneficial in further improving technology to deal with the challenges ahead through the pandemic. Rapid innovation also seems to lead to optimism among politicians, in particular with respect to track-and-trace applications. When new interventions/tools are designed, as in the context of COVID-19, we must remain cautious and realise the barriers of implementing them. It is often worth using already developed and proven technologies instead of constantly striving for innovation. Importantly, and referring to the seminal paper (Eysenbach, 2001), eHealth's use has advantages classifiable on topics like efficiency, enhancing quality, equity, and empowerment; however, it should be implemented with caution considering issues of data protection and privacy.

Technology interventions are needed to prevent the spread of COVID-19 at a significant scale. For instance, videoconferencing can facilitate social distancing. Technology can also be of great help, either when informing the wider public and targeting prevention or helping people to cope with specific problems that may have risen due to COVID-19. Kelders and Howard (2018) describe the advantages of technology under the heading 'Technology as a persuader' and refer to (Fogg, 2002). They state: 'Technology offers specific opportunities to be an influential persuader with its persistence, anonymity, ability to deal with large amounts of data, uses of many modalities, its scalability and its being able to be everywhere' (p. 65). Technology has added value because of these qualities; it will, for example, not get tired of intervening, and it can help tackling sensitive issues that might be at stake with COVID-19, such as handling data on a possible infection. The significant advantage though, referring to the public health challenges related to COVID-19, is that technology is capable of delivering behaviour change programs at a large scale, reaching out to the wide population. To understand today's *digital revolution,* it is helpful to familiarise yourself with its evolution looking at the three identified layers on which technology is used to improve health: human elements, technology foundations, and interaction capabilities. In order to design useful and user-friendly technology, also during COVID-19 pandemic, it is crucial to build digital health solutions based on behaviour change theories and consider human-computer-interactions that are largely underpinned by psychological notions.

In this chapter the authors elaborate on what kind of technologies can be distinguished that can then form a basis for building behavioural interventions. They discern: (a) cognitive computing (systems that mimic the human brain – like the IBM system *Watson*, a question-answering computer system, High, 2012), (b) embodied conversational agents in which the technology can support the users through voice modality (e.g., with feedback messages to patients/users) (Van

Pinxteren et al., 2020), (c) virtual reality, and (d) wearable technology for self-tracking. These various technologies can be used to build new, or refine existing, systems in relation to prevention (as aforementioned the track-and-trace applications) and also interventions focusing on specific health outcomes. For instance, COVID-19 patient fatigue is often mentioned as a significant disturbing symptom in the long-term. Systems with fully automatic application, like the Untire App (Spahrkäs et al., 2020), built for use in cancer survivors, may have application to support COVID-19 patients struggling with fatigue.

Finally, the authors address the issue of the development of (eHealth) technology, describing Artificial Intelligence, which deals with how the computer is programmed to (re)act in similar manner as human beings. They elaborate on machine learning, natural language processing, and neural networks. In this chapter Kelders and Howard point out that social scientists need to have a basic knowledge of technology. They also give a short overview of the developmental steps taken in designing and producing eHealth programs, describing the critical and essential development steps within the umbrella term *agile development*. This term refers to the process in which the software is developed in small steps and tested, again and again, while involving stakeholders from different perspectives. This also relates to the difficult issue of wide-scale implementation and the need to involve several stakeholders, in particular the users.

The fourth chapter by Deborah Lupton is about 'The lived experience of digital health'. This chapter encourages and inspires us to think about when and how to use technology, and what to consider when designing technology for use in a health context. The chapter explains how technology can be used and incorporated into everyday life. The author provides examples of the use of technology in various environmental settings, and with different goals in patients groups (like HIV/AIDS, diabetes and patients on dialysis who use technology for self-management tasks) and in healthy individuals (e.g., when making use of self-tracking to optimise health status).

The author describes the online platforms used by patients, which can be very helpful, for example, for patients with an illness that can be associated with stigma (like HIV/AIDS). We already know that – depending on cultural context – patients infected with COVID-19 can be confronted with rejection from within their community. These kinds of platforms enable patients to share emotions and obtain support; although, at the same time, they may lead to highly normative opinions which may have a countereffect on the emotional state of a person sharing a personal story. Technology may also have both positive and negative outcomes, where healthcare workers strive to empower patients in sharing medical data with the patients. Some patients do not want to access personal and sensitive information online, and choose to have first a face-to-face contact with their doctor. Popular opinion is that the elderly avoid the use of technology; however, we have to be aware that young people may also not support its use. Digital self-management tools can positively support management of patients' disease, but also have several complexities associated with their use. Deborah Lupton raises the critical issue that those who develop and try to implement technology (such as designers, policymakers, healthcare workers) 'often do not recognize the shifting and heterogeneous lifeworld's which the devices enter' (p 109). The author also mentions that people do not merely use technology or reject it, but quite often move between these positions. Hence, the entire chapter emphasises the importance of stakeholder involvement to improve understanding of optimal design and delivery of technology to encourage optimal use.

In the fifth chapter, by Andrew Prestwich, Jared B. Kenworthy and Mark Conner, the reader is introduced to 'Environment- and policy-based approaches to health behavior change'. During the pandemic, it has become apparent that environment and policy shape how we live our lives and behavioural scientists have an opportunity to influence COVID-19 policies. For example, in the Netherlands, a team of virologists and doctors that advises the government on how to best respond to COVID-19 has been expanded to include behavioural scientists. This group advises on the best options for potential behavioural interventions, how to communicate the measures, and how to reach minority groups to protect them from the virus. We also see similar initiatives in other countries, such as the UK (e.g., Bonell et al., 2020). Considering that policy is often insufficiently informed by the science of behaviour, current developments rooted in evidence-based behaviour change insights from behavioural experts are positive.

In this chapter the authors examine the role of environmental factors and policies that influence health behaviours, and provide relevant examples including: *structural*, such as a lack of suitable exercise facilities, and *personal*, such as a lack of financial resources to buy healthy food. Similar environmental barriers can be relevant in the COVID-19 pandemic, when the community may lack structural resources, for instance, the healthcare system being under-resourced and overwhelmed due to the high number of inpatients (Grasselli et al., 2020). People in the community may lack personal resources, for instance adequate handwashing facilities, face masks, and protective clothing, or not be able to stay at home (e.g., due to work demands) (Truelove et al., 2020). In this chapter the authors consider direct, mediated, and moderated effects by which environmental factors may influence human behaviour. They refer to nudge theory and choice architecture as examples of the introduction of environmental change to influence and shape human behaviour. For instance, during the pandemic we are being 'nudged' to wash our hands, with posters placed in bathrooms to remind us about the COVID-19 risk and the importance of proper handwashing. In supermarkets and shops, stickers placed on the floor mark safe physical distance (in most countries 1.5 meters) between customers to prevent virus spread. In terms of choice architecture, our choices are often shaped by the environment; for instance, the accessibility of staircases will determine use of the stairs or lifts; the place where healthy products are positioned in the shops in relation to the unhealthy snack will affect which products we select.

In this chapter the authors also examine the research on how changes in the environment may produce changes in psychological cognitions, such as social norms or intentions that, in turn, impact behaviour. In the times of the COVID-19 pandemic our environment has changed dramatically and instantly, as new norms and measures were introduced and scaled across the society to prevent virus spread. We are encouraged to stay at home, to social distance, and to self-isolate if we are exhibiting any symptoms. Our attitudes also changed radically. At the start many of us did not perceive COVID-19 as a real threat, but with time and access to relevant information, most people changed their attitudes and perceptions of the virus and the risks posed to the society. The authors of the chapter also reflect on the effects of public policy-based solutions and social marketing approaches to change behaviour. Social marketing is key in the promotion of protective behaviours during COVID-19 (Bonell et al., 2020), and campaigns were established across the world to slow and stop the spread of the virus. We are encouraged to protect ourselves and to protect others, and the following chapter on 'self-as-doer identity' can support us to do so.

In Chapter 6 Amanda M. Brouwer looks at 'self-as-doer identity' and health behaviour change. The self-as-doer identity is described in terms of perceiving yourself as the doer of behaviours that are leading to the successful enactment and maintenance of health goals. This theory links self-concept to behaviour in order to conceptualise oneself as the doer of that behaviour to support behaviour change and maintenance, similarly to the process of reinvention theory (Ogden & Hills, 2008). Adopting and maintaining healthy lifestyle behaviours is key to optimal health (Kwasnicka et al., 2016) and self-as-doer identity supports long-term health behaviour change. The research reviewed in this chapter supports the self-as-doer theory demonstrating that doer identification predicts health behaviour change and maintenance. Researchers have identified several health behaviours described in this chapter that contribute to better health outcomes and the reduction of disease risk. Specific behaviours described here that are widely encouraged by policy makers and public health experts during the COVID-19 pandemic are: regular physical activity, a healthy diet, and limited alcohol consumption. Engaging in a combination of these health behaviours will further improve health and reduce health risks.

Similarly, researchers suggest that physical activity is now particularly useful to fight against the mental and physical consequences of the COVID-19 quarantine, especially for the elderly (Jiménez-Pavón et al., 2020). Encouraging physical activity at home, and physical activity and shopping for food supplies are the only allowable exceptions for leaving the house during the pandemic (e.g., in the UK, in Poland, in the Netherlands, even during the stricter stages of the lockdown). Furthermore, compelling evidence showed that dietary habits are affected by stress and emotional disturbance, and elevated distress is associated with unhealthy dietary patterns and relatively poor diet quality (Naja & Hamadeh, 2020). Stress is also a prominent risk factor for the onset and maintenance of alcohol misuse (Clay & Parker, 2020). The self-as-doer identity theory is likely to be useful for creating behavioural change in terms of physical activity, healthy eating, and avoidance of excessive alcohol consumption for promoting the maintenance of that change during the pandemic. To understand the self-as-doer identity, two studies, one on physical activity and one on diet, are discussed in this chapter.

This chapter can motivate the reader to change self-perceptions and to change their own activity and dietary habits during the pandemic, and to maintain these health changes post COVID-19.

The final, very brief chapter by Ken J. Rotenberg titled '*Trust and health: The road to wellness*' emphasises the importance of trusting medical professionals. Again, very relevant during COVID-19 pandemic is the notion of trusting healthcare professionals to provide us with adequate tests and treatment if infected with the virus. In this chapter the author focuses on trusting physicians, doctors, and nurses, from the psychological research perspective. Although there is a broader domain of medical trust (e.g., trust in leaders, systems) that is not covered in this chapter. The author here emphasises that a number of studies show that adults' and children's trust beliefs in healthcare professionals are associated with successful medical treatment. The studies show that patients have better treatment results when they trust their doctors. They also are more likely to have better adherence to medication, better satisfaction with the healthcare received, stronger intention to follow the healthcare professional's advice, and even better symptoms improvement. So, it seems that trust of healthcare professionals is crucial, and may improve several medical outcomes.

The notion of trust in healthcare professionals during the COVID-19 pandemic, with the mass-spreading of misinformation and social media promoting 'fake news', may undermine healthcare professionals' advice (O'Connor & Murphy, 2020). With the use of new technologies to protect health, the World Health Organization has confronted fake news by offering a WhatsApp service to eliminate misinformation and to provide relevant updates. Evidence also shows that healthcare professionals can stop the spread of misinformation by rebutting misleading health information on social media and providing accurate advice (O'Connor & Murphy, 2020). At the end of this chapter, the author asks: 'Are there consequences of being too trusting in the medical profession?' and provides a suggestion for forming a patient–healthcare professional working relationship. This relationship needs to be based on empathy, trust, and shared decision making. This chapter reviews the research showing that general trust and trust in healthcare professionals (and even trust in romantic partners) are associated with better health. Facing COVID-19 pandemic in times of rapid access to information and widespread misinformation, it is important that we trust our healthcare professionals, and seek accurate advice. We need to challenge information given and build relations with healthcare professionals that are based on trust and mutual respect, while understanding different perspectives, backgrounds, and attitudes. We are all in this together.

Conclusions

Psychology helps answer many of the topical questions that many of us are asking ourselves now: How do we change ingrained behaviour such as regular handwashing, physical distancing, and staying at home? How can we motivate people to be attentive to symptoms, show willingness to get tested, and comply with quarantine rules? How can we help people to cope with the stress of a pandemic – including dealing with loneliness as a result of physical isolation? How can we develop interventions and programs using technology to help people deal with the pandemic and recover afterwards? How do the population perceive newly introduced measures, and respond and adjust to these measures? This book attempts to answer these questions in the time of the COVID-19 pandemic. The book aims to introduce certain aspects of psychology: (1) health, behaviour change, and well-being; (2) dealing with stress and changing the environment; and (3) making use of technology. The knowledge offered can be helpful to address the challenges of the COVID-19 pandemic and can be viewed in two ways. On one hand, much can be done to support primary prevention, to prevent people from contracting the virus. On the other hand, the knowledge can be used to deal with stressful situations and recover after illness. This book provides psychological perspective on the COVID-19 pandemic and hopefully will guide the reader through the new realities we are facing today.

References

Anderson, M., Mckee, M., & Mossialos, E. (2020). Developing a sustainable exit strategy for COVID-19: Health, economic and public policy implications. *Journal of the Royal Society of Medicine*, *113*(5), 176–178.

Bonell, C., Michie, S., Reicher, S., West, R., Bear, L., Yardley, L., Curtis, V., Amlôt, R., & Rubin, G. J. (2020). Harnessing behavioural science in public health campaigns to maintain 'social distancing'in response to the COVID-19 pandemic: Key principles. *J Epidemiol Community Health.*

Clay, J. M., & Parker, M. O. (2020). Alcohol use and misuse during the COVID-19 pandemic: A potential public health crisis? *The Lancet Public Health*, *5*(5), e259.

Eysenbach, G. (2001). What is e-health? *Journal of Medical Internet Research*, *3*(2), e20. https://doi.org/10.2196/jmir.3.2.e20

Fogg, B. J. (2002). Persuasive technology: Using computers to change what we think and do. *Ubiquity*, *2002*(December), 2. https://doi.org/10.1145/764008.763957

Grasselli, G., Pesenti, A., & Cecconi, M. (2020). Critical care utilization for the COVID-19 outbreak in Lombardy, Italy: Early experience and forecast during an emergency response. *Jama*, *323*(16), 1545–1546.

Hellewell, J., Abbott, S., Gimma, A., Bosse, N. I., Jarvis, C. I., Russell, T. W., Munday, J. D., Kucharski, A. J., Edmunds, W. J., & Sun, F. (2020). Feasibility of controlling COVID-19 outbreaks by isolation of cases and contacts. *The Lancet Global Health.*

High, R. (2012). The era of cognitive systems: An inside look at IBM Watson and how it works. *IBM Corporation, Redbooks*, 1–16.

Howarth, C., Bryant, P., Corner, A., Fankhauser, S., Gouldson, A., Whitmarsh, L., & Willis, R. (2020). Building a social mandate for climate action: Lessons from COVID-19. *Environmental and Resource Economics*, 1–9.

Jee, Y. (2020). WHO International Health Regulations Emergency Committee for the COVID-19 outbreak. *Epidemiology and Health*, *42*.

Jiménez-Pavón, D., Carbonell-Baeza, A., & Lavie, C. J. (2020). Physical exercise as therapy to fight against the mental and physical consequences of COVID-19 quarantine: Special focus in older people. *Progress in Cardiovascular Diseases.*

Jovančević, A., & Milićević, N. (2020). Optimism-pessimism, conspiracy theories and general trust as factors contributing to COVID-19 related behavior – A cross-cultural study. *Personality and Individual Differences*, *167*, 110216. https://doi.org/10.1016/j.paid.2020.110216

Kwasnicka, D., Dombrowski, S. U., White, M., & Sniehotta, F. (2016). Theoretical explanations for maintenance of behaviour change: A systematic review of behaviour theories. *Health Psychology Review*, *10*(3), 277–296.

McKee, M., & Stuckler, D. (2020). If the world fails to protect the economy, COVID-19 will damage health not just now but also in the future. *Nature Medicine*, *26*(5), 640–642.

Naja, F., & Hamadeh, R. (2020). Nutrition amid the COVID-19 pandemic: A multi-level framework for action. *European Journal of Clinical Nutrition*, 1–5.

Nicola, M., Alsafi, Z., Sohrabi, C., Kerwan, A., Al-Jabir, A., Iosifidis, C., Agha, M., & Agha, R. (2020). The socio-economic implications of the coronavirus and COVID-19 pandemic: A review. *International Journal of Surgery*.

O'Connor, C., & Murphy, M. (2020). Going viral: Doctors must tackle fake news in the covid-19 pandemic. *Bmj*, *24*(369), m1587.

Ogden, J., & Hills, L. (2008). Understanding sustained behavior change: The role of life crises and the process of reinvention. *Health:*, *12*(4), 419–437.

Park, T., Ju, I., Ohs, J. E., & Hinsley, A. (2020). Optimistic bias and preventive behavioral engagement in the context of COVID-19. *Research in Social and Administrative Pharmacy*, S1551741120306811. https://doi.org/10.1016/j.sapharm.2020.06.004

Polizzi, C., Lynn, S. J., & Perry, A. (2020). Stress and coping in the time of COVID-19: Pathways to resilience and recovery. *Clinical Neuropsychiatry*, *17*(2).

Sachs, J. D., Horton, R., Bagenal, J., Amor, Y. B., Caman, O. K., & Lafortune, G. (2020). The Lancet COVID-19 Commission. *The Lancet*.

Spahrkäs, S. S., Looijmans, A., Sanderman, R., & Hagedoorn, M. (2020). Beating Cancer-Related Fatigue with the "Untire" Mobile App: Results from a Waiting-List Randomized Controlled Trial. *Psycho-Oncology*, pon.5492. https://doi.org/10.1002/pon.5492

Truelove, S., Abrahim, O., Altare, C., Lauer, S. A., Grantz, K. H., Azman, A. S., & Spiegel, P. (2020). The potential impact of COVID-19 in refugee camps in Bangladesh and beyond: A modeling study. *PLoS Medicine*, *17*(6), e1003144.

Van Bavel, J. J., Baicker, K., Boggio, P. S., Capraro, V., Cichocka, A., Cikara, M., Crockett, M. J., Crum, A. J., Douglas, K. M., & Druckman, J. N. (2020). Using social and behavioural science to support COVID-19 pandemic response. *Nature Human Behaviour*, 1–12.

van Gemert-Pijnen, L., Kelders, S. M., Kip, H., & Sanderman, R. (2018). *eHealth research, theory and development: A multi-disciplinary approach*. Routledge.

Van Pinxteren, M. M., Pluymaekers, M., & Lemmink, J. G. (2020). Human-like communication in conversational agents: A literature review and research agenda. *Journal of Service Management*.

Wang, C., Pan, R., Wan, X., Tan, Y., Xu, L., Ho, C. S., & Ho, R. C. (2020). Immediate psychological responses and associated factors during the initial stage of the 2019 coronavirus disease (COVID-19) epidemic among the general population in China. *International Journal of Environmental Research and Public Health*, *17*(5), 1729.

Whitelaw, S., Mamas, M. A., Topol, E., & Van Spall, H. G. (2020). Applications of digital technology in COVID-19 pandemic planning and response. *The Lancet Digital Health*.

Wosik, J., Fudim, M., Cameron, B., Gellad, Z. F., Cho, A., Phinney, D., Curtis, S., Roman, M., Poon, E. G., & Ferranti, J. (2020). Telehealth Transformation: COVID-19 and the rise of Virtual Care. *Journal of the American Medical Informatics Association, 27*(6), 957–962.

Xiao, Y., & Torok, M. E. (2020). Taking the right measures to control COVID-19. *The Lancet Infectious Diseases, 20*(5), 523–524.

CHAPTER 1

Emotional Health and Well-Being

This chapter was first published in *Health Psychology* 3ed and cross-referencing relates to chapters in the original volume. Please visit www.routledge.com/9781138201309 for more information about the book

Chapter Outline

Chapter Objectives

After reading this chapter you will be able to:

1. Identify and define four major models of health and well-being.
2. Compare and contrast the concept of well-being in the four models.
3. Define *positive psychology*.
4. Identify three studies that demonstrate the beneficial effects of positive affect on health.
5. Identify and explain two criticisms of the positive psychology movement.
6. Describe three major types of traditional medicine.
7. Compare and contrast traditional versus modern medicine.

OPENING STORY: ANGELITA

Miguel was getting worried. For the past three months, his wife, Angelita, seemed inexplicably sad. Usually cheerful, talkative, and energetic, Angelita had become increasingly quiet and weepy. She complained of frequent headaches and spent hours alone in her garden. The only activity she seemed to enjoy was cooking. For example, when cooking her favorite foods from her hometown of La Paz, Mexico, Angelita could be heard singing for hours. But during dinner, she would become quiet. She would feel her stomach begin to "churn" and then excuse herself from the table.

Miguel encouraged Angelita to see her doctor. He hoped that a physical exam would uncover the problem. Angelita's doctor, however, found no viral or bacterial infection and no other physical explanations for the headaches. The doctor believed that Angelita's symptoms were rooted in emotional problems but was uncertain of the cause. He suggested that she come back in one week if there was no improvement in her condition, and he would refer her to someone who could help address what he suspected were emotional problems.

Angelita decided not to return to her doctor. She believed that because he had no idea what was wrong he could be of no help. Instead, she phoned her mother, Carmen, and told her about her current health problems. Carmen, who still lived in La Paz, convinced her daughter to come to Mexico for a week of rest and relaxation. In truth, Carmen wanted Angelita to see the village ***curandero,*** *a traditional healer who practiced a form of medicine called* ***curanderismo,*** *found in many Latin American countries. Curanderismo is a holistic approach to health that treats a person's material, spiritual, and psychic health in addition to his or her physical needs (Trotter, 2001). Carmen believed that curanderismo was preferable to modern health practices, especially when dealing with emotional or other nonphysical health issues.*

Carmen notified the curandero, and, as is the custom, the curandero agreed to visit Angelita at home. He came the day after Angelita arrived and spent several hours talking with her. Angelita remembered that the curandero's father was the village healer when she was a child. It appeared that in the time that had passed, the healing gift, referred to as "el don," was passed to the son. After talking with Angelita, the curandero gave her an herb tea to drink and rubbed a salve over her temples and forehead. He said he would return to check on Angelita in two days.

On his second visit, the curandero brought more herbs and made another tea. He then asked Angelita about her adjustment to her new home and neighborhood in Nashville, Tennessee. When he learned that Angelita could not find in Nashville the same herbs and spices used for cooking and for teas that she used in Mexico, he gave her extra to take with her when she returned. He also gave her a small pillow filled with strong scents.

Within a week of returning to Nashville, Angelita began feeling better. She seemed happier and appeared more energetic, much like her "old" self. Because she no longer complained of headaches, she was more social and no longer needed long periods of solitude. Angelita called her mother to report the changes, and Carmen immediately relayed the news to the curandero. The curandero replied simply that Angelita needed to reconnect spiritually to her home and culture. He believed that the Mexican herbs he gave Angelita would make her spirit more content while away from her home. ■

Traditional medicines like curanderismo may have originated several millennia ago, but they are still used throughout the world today. As we saw in the opening story, some people use traditional medicines in addition to or in lieu of Western, medical approaches. Recall that Angelita sought the assistance of the curandero only after seeking assistance from her doctor in Nashville. Her mother, however, preferred to use curanderismo as a first or only option.

Using traditional medicines, the curandero determined (or diagnosed, if you prefer) that Angelita's physical symptoms were caused largely by spiritual and emotional health problems, a longing for the familiar. Yet Angelita's doctor in Nashville, who uses Western medical techniques, also concluded that her problem was not physical in origin. In fact, if pressed, the doctor might have suggested that Angelita was suffering from a bout of homesickness, a type of ***psychosomatic illness*** with emotional or psychological underlying causes. Thus, both traditional and Western medicinal practitioners concluded that Angelita experienced an emotional health problem, even though they differed somewhat as to the cause. In the opening story we introduce one theme of the current chapter: the contrasting and complementary practices of traditional versus Western medicine. We will explore the similarities and differences between both forms of medicine, focusing specifically on their treatment of emotional health issues.

The opening story also illustrates the effects of emotional factors on overall health outcomes. Specifically, Angelita's story reminds us that emotions contribute to our physical state. Thus, in this chapter, we also explore the role of emotional health on overall well-being. In the process, we will identify the contributions of health psychologists to understanding emotions as a health determinant.

We begin our exploration of emotional health by examining four models used currently in research and practice in the field of health psychology: the biomedical model, the biopsychosocial model, the wellness model, and the ecological (sometimes called social ecological) model. The models were developed and tested in the 20th century largely in Western cultures and therefore represent a modern day view of health.

In Section II, we explore a new topic called positive psychology. Positive psychology proposes that to understand human outcomes we must identify and examine all contributing factors, positive as well as negative. Included in this concept is a focus on health-enhancing emotional factors that can lead to good health outcomes. According to this view, the positive emotions, experiences, and personal characteristics that contribute to healthy outcomes have been largely overlooked in psychology. Proponents of positive psychology suggest that if we omit the study of "normal" healthy states, we cannot fully understand health.

Finally, in Section III, we explore a sample of traditional medicines, including Chinese traditional medicine, folk medicines that include *curanderismo* and *sangoma,* and a brief overview of Native American healing practices. Again, our focus when reviewing traditional medicines is principally to understand the similarities and differences between traditional and Western medicines as well as the relationship between emotions and overall well-being as explained by these two perspectives.

After reading this chapter, you will be able to identify and explain four models of health currently used to diagnose outcomes, to explain the role of emotions on individual health outcomes, to identify the central concepts of positive psychology and its contribution to our understanding of health outcomes, and to compare the treatment of emotional health in Western and traditional medicines.

Consider two important points before proceeding. First, you will notice that some of the health models use the term ***well-being*** to characterize an individual's overall state of health. As noted in Chapter 1, An Interdisciplinary View of Health, well-being describes the state of the body (physical), the mind (psychological), the spirit, and social relations (emotions). It offers a holistic view of health similar to the ecological model, with one distinction. The ecological model does not specifically address spiritual health. It does, however, include physical environmental factors as well as health systems and health policy determinants. Because well-being incorporates many of the same determinants found in the biopsychosocial model, we will use this term rather than *health* to characterize a person's overall condition (physical, psychological, emotional, and social). When applicable, we will add to this concept the effects of the physical and psychological environment, health systems, and health policy on health outcomes to explain the ecological model.

Second, and equally as important, by using the term *well-being* we are reminded that a thorough study of health integrates the emotional and psychological states of an individual. It further supports the inclusion of health psychologists into the practice of and research on health.

SECTION I. FOUR MODELS OF WELL-BEING

Biomedical Model

The first formal, Western model of well-being, here meaning a model supported by scientific inquiry and empirical study, is the ***biomedical model***. In favor since the early 20th century, the biomedical model proposed that health is the absence of disease or dysfunction. Using this definition as a starting point, *disease* was defined as an abnormality, specifically a dysfunction of or deviation in a body organ or other body structure (Engel, 2002; Wade & Halligan, 2004). Thus, according to the biomedical model, a person who is in good health will be free of any abnormal biological changes in or functions of the body, whereas someone in "bad" or ill health will experience a change in the body system or functions. Furthermore, when diseases occur, this model suggests that locating and eradicating the illness will restore a person to good health.

As we saw in Chapter 1, An Interdisciplinary View of Health, a wholly physiologically based concept of health is consistent with some earlier beliefs. For example, the Cnidians in 500 BCE in Greece and the Roman philosopher and physician Galen in 200 CE believed that physical maladies determined an individual's health status. Research suggests that the early views were enhanced and supported by later studies performed in the 1880s by Robert Koch of Germany and by Louis Pasteur of France (Cantor, 2000; Checkland et al., 2008).

In separate, some say rival, studies, Koch established that "invisible germs carried contagions." In support of that assertion, Koch identified specific microorganisms that caused diseases such as anthrax and tuberculosis (Tan & Berman, 2008). The irrefutable association between a specific organism and a specific disease convinced many Western scientists that illnesses were indeed caused only by microorganisms.

Pasteur's work, which pioneered the use of vaccines to prevent infectious diseases (see Chapter 3, Global Communicable and Chronic Disease) (Pasteur, Chamberlain, & Roux, 2002), further supported the germ theory of disease. Thus, it appeared that Koch's discovery of the relationship between microorganisms and disease and Pasteur's discovery of vaccines that protect individuals from such microorganisms (thereby ensuring good health) explained the origins of illness. These two seminal studies appear to have led to the development of the biomedical model of health (Checkland et al., 2008).

LIMITATIONS OF THE BIOMEDICAL MODEL To be certain, science supports the association between microorganisms and disease, the central tenet of the biomedical model. Unfortunately, the assertion that only physical agents cause illnesses is also a limitation of the model. Other limitations include a problem-oriented approach to health and wellness and a broad, perhaps overbroad, definition of illness. We review each limitation briefly here.

The belief that only physiological determinants cause illness presents, as Engel (2002) suggests, a "culturally specific perspective about diseases," somewhat like a Western-culture version of folk medicine.

Past and current models of health, in addition to current research, suggest that microorganisms are only one of several factors that influence health outcomes. By focusing on the physical causes of illness, the biomedical model overlooks emotional or psychological determinants that also influence well-being. We explain the specific role of non-physiological factors on health later in this chapter.

A second limitation is the problem-oriented focus of the biomedical model. It proposes that a change in normal bodily functions that results in a deviation from or dysfunction of the body signals a problem to be rectified. But consider this: Would someone with a hearing impairment or someone who is deaf be considered ill because of his or her dysfunctional auditory system? Probably not. Few people equate dysfunction with an illness. Indeed, some individuals who are hearing impaired may characterize their limitations as a disability, but few would consider themselves ill. Yet, according to the biomedical model, a dysfunctional auditory system would be considered an illness.

Even the assumption that physical symptoms are clear indications of an illness or disease can be challenged. Let us return to our opening story. Angelita experienced physical symptoms, prompting her to seek medical care. But, according to the biomedical model's definition of health, she was not ill. There was no underlying viral or bacteriological disease that caused her symptoms. Nothing was broken. Still, it was evident that Angelita was not in a state of well-being. Clearly, she was experiencing some type of health problem—just not the sort recognized by the biomedical model.

In addition, consider this: Some illnesses can occur independent of symptoms. Hypertension, a heart-related disease that we will explore in Chapter 9, Cardiovascular Disease, is nicknamed "the silent killer" because it often develops with no observable, here meaning external, symptoms. Similarly, individuals may often be unaware that they have been infected with a deadly human immunodeficiency virus because it, too, often carries no noticeable external symptoms for the first eight to ten years. Thus, in some cases, external symptoms of an illness can appear without evidence of an underlying disease (like Angelita's problem). In other instances, a disease may indeed be present (like hypertension or HIV), but show no visible or external symptom, especially in the early stages of illness.

To summarize, the biomedical model defines *dysfunctionality* as an illness and interprets physiological symptoms as signs of the illness. But the biologically based model presents a limited definition of illness that can include a range of dysfunctions not usually classified as an illness. For example, a person who is deaf has a dysfunctional auditory system. Yet few would determine that a deaf person has an illness. Current research suggests that a more precise yet also in some ways broader definition of health may be more accurate and may include the emotional, psychological, and, for some, spiritual determinants of well-being (Nikelly, 2005).

Let us consider one point before moving on. It is important to restate that a broad definition of health and well-being is not new. Recall that in Chapter 1, An Interdisciplinary View of Health, we briefly reviewed the health practices and beliefs of civilizations including ancient Greeks (specifically Aesculapius and Hippocrates), Chinese civilizations, Native Americans, and the Sans and Yoruba cultures in southern and western Africa. All of these civilizations embraced a holistic or an ecological view of health that included the emotional, physical, psychological, environmental, and, for some, the spiritual well-being of the individual.

In more recent times, research by Sigmund Freud in the 1890s reaffirmed a broad concept of health, one that included emotional and psychological factors. Specifically, Freud suggested that many of the physical illnesses described by his patients were, in fact, linked to psychological causes. When the psychological problems were addressed, he noted that the physical symptoms were also resolved without direct treatment. Contemporary health and behavioral medicine furthered Freud's version of the mind–body connection by establishing the field of psychosomatic medicine. This new discipline abolished the separation of the mind and body proposed in earlier versions of Western medicine (Mizrachi, 2001) and reintroduced a holistic concept of well-being. Thus our brief review of health in Chapter 1 that highlighted examples of holistic and ecological health models set the stage for further exploration of the role of emotions on health in Western and traditional medicines. The biopsychosocial, wellness, and social ecological models are examples of such models.

Biopsychosocial Model

Sometimes referred to as a ***holistic health model,*** the ***biopsychosocial model*** proposed by Engel (2002) supports the belief, endorsed by many in health psychology, that well-being is determined by biological (*bio*), psychological (*psycho*), and sociological (*social*) factors. The psychological influences on health include emotions, health behaviors, personality traits, and social support systems and their effects on emotional health (Lazarus & Folkman, 1987; Ryan & Deci, 2000; Salovey, Rothman, Detweiler, & Steward, 2000), while sociological factors include familial, cultural, and community factors. We examine some of the psychological and sociological factors in turn.

PSYCHOLOGICAL FACTOR #1: EMOTIONS We noted earlier that the relationship between health and emotions was proposed many centuries earlier. ***Hippocrates,*** sometimes called the father of clinical medicine, is often credited with pioneering the interaction of emotions and health in Western medicine. He believed that an imbalance in any one of four bodily fluids, called ***humors,*** could lead to illnesses (Salovey et al., 2000). The important part is that the illnesses he identified were, in fact, emotional. For example, Hippocrates believed that an imbalance of black bile, one type of body fluids, would lead to sadness or melancholy, while an imbalance of yellow bile, another fluid, led to anger. We will see later in the chapter that traditional medicines also defined well-being as a balance between emotional, physical, social, and environmental forces.

The concept presented by Hippocrates that links health and emotions is supported by current research, although the details have changed considerably. Current studies show that emotions can affect our physiological well-being through two primary pathways: our immune system and our behaviors.

Emotions and the Immune System Rabin and colleagues (1989) suggest that one way that emotions affect our immune system is through the nerve fibers in our bodies. The fibers connect with the ***central nervous system (CNS),*** the "control center" for our body or, biologically speaking, the brain and the brain stem (see Figure 6.1).

The nerve fibers act like cables carrying information from our ***receptors*** (skin, muscles, and other sites), to our central nervous system (CNS). It may help to think of the neuron cables as the hardware needed to communicate. The actual message, however, is carried by **neurotransmitters** that travel within the cables. When sending messages from a receptor site—such as the skin—to the brain, a neurotransmitter is triggered at the receptor site and passed along from neuron to neuron via the axons and dendrites until the message reaches the processing center of the brain. ***Dendrites,*** from the Greek word *dendron,* meaning tree, are branchlike structures that extend from the cell body and receive the message from other cells. Once the message is received, the ***axon,*** another nerve fiber that extends from the cell body, carries the message to neighboring cells (see Figure 6.2).

The nerve cables that carry messages are categorized as either afferent or efferent nerve fibers. The ***afferent nerve fibers*** carry information to the CNS (the brain and the spinal cord) from the receptor sites.

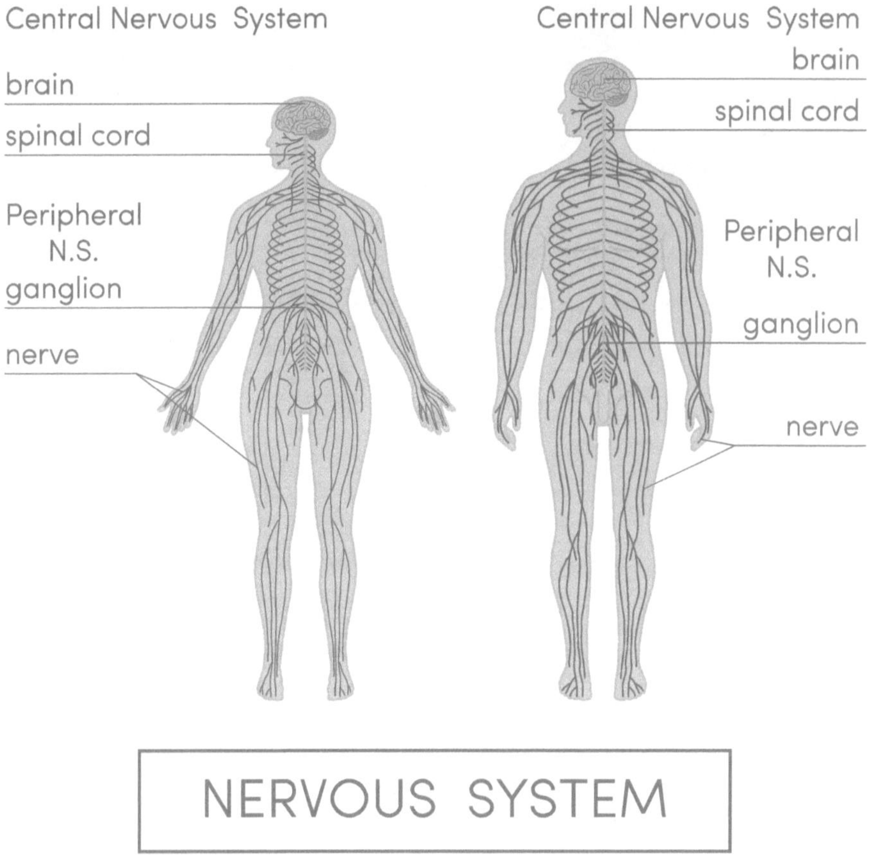

FIGURE 6.1 The Central Nervous System, Brain, and Brain Stem.

Source: note replacement pending

For example, if a person touches a sharp object, the afferent nerves may send a sensory signal from the fingers (the receptor site) to the brain or spinal cord for processing and interpretation. The ***efferent nerve fibers,*** on the other hand, carry information from the CNS to the periphery of the body to coordinate the response. Using the same example of touching a sharp object, the brain might send a signal of pain or discomfort to the receptor site (hand) that results in the person withdrawing his or her hand from the sharp object.

Impact of Emotions on Health Now that we understand the basic structure of the body's neurological communication system, we can examine the effects of our emotions on the communication process and hence on our overall well-being. There are a number of research studies on stress that help demonstrate this effect (Cohen, Tyrrell, & Smith, 1991, 1993; Dusek & Benson, 2009; Jacobs, 2001; Kiecolt-Glaser &

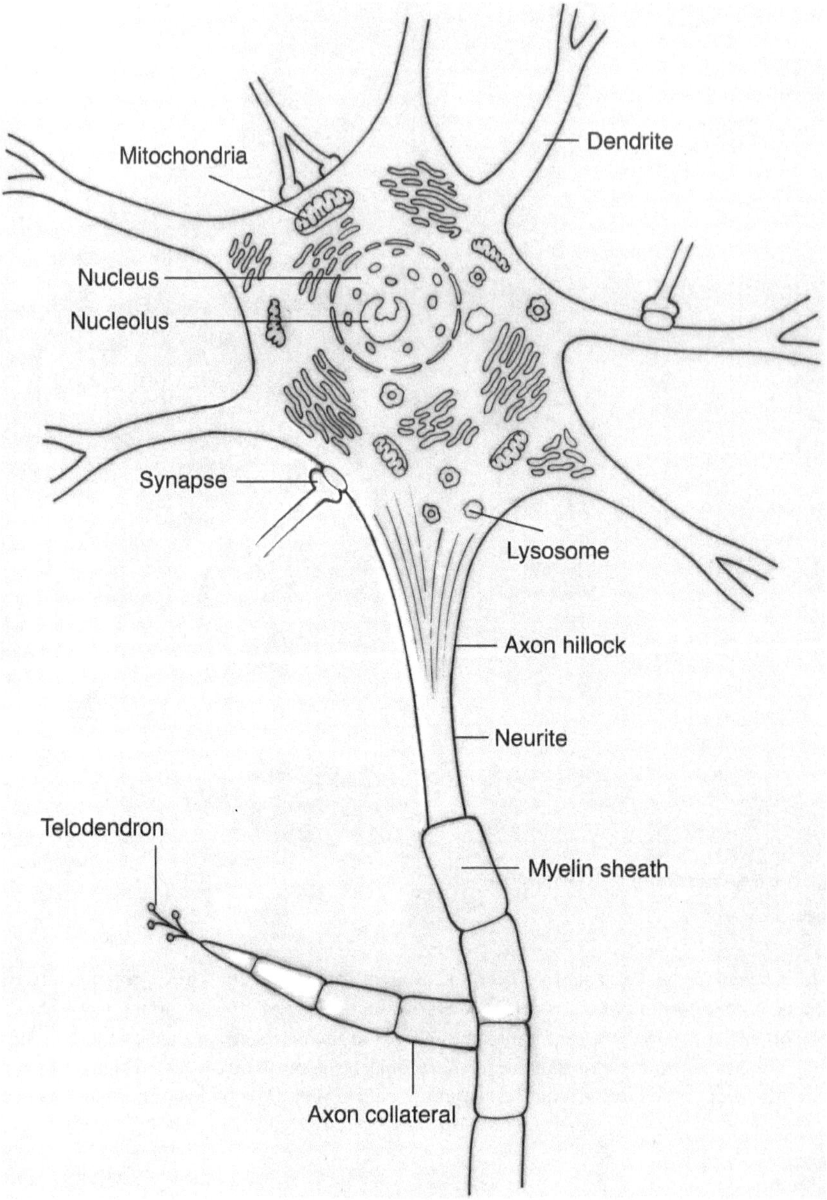

FIGURE 6.2 Structure of a Human Cell.

Source: CO 172586-Illustration_of_motor_neuron_Sci photolibrary,jpg

Glaser, 1988; Williams & Williams, 1993). In studies examining the effects of stress on the body's ***immune system,*** here meaning the body's defense against illness-producing microorganisms, Cohen (2005) found that stress may influence the production of ***hormones,*** another type of chemical message released by cells in our body that, in turn, affect the immune system.

How do hormones influence health outcomes? We review stress and the immune systems in Chapter 7, Stress and Coping, and in greater detail in Chapter 8, Psychoneuroimmunology. But for now, one example of the relationship between stress and the immune system is seen through the role of ***epinephrine,*** a stress hormone that helps to suppress the immune system. Suppressing or "turning down" the body's immune system decreases the body's ability to fight foreign or disease-carrying microorganisms and increases the risk of contracting a disease. Thus, if an individual experiences high levels or extended periods of stress, that person's body may increase production of epinephrine and signal the brain to suppress the immune system. A person who contracts a viral or bacterial illness while his or her immune system is functioning at lower levels will be less able to ward off the illness.

Applied health psychology research that tests the proposed link between emotions and illnesses similarly reports a correlation between emotions and health. For example, research by Schulz, Martire, Beach, and Scheier (2005) and Schulz and colleagues (2000) established a link between depression and mortality. In their study of approximately 5,200 participants aged 65 or older, individuals with depressive symptoms were 25% more likely to die within six years than were individuals with considerably lower levels of depression (Schulz et al., 2000). In essence, their study suggests that an emotional factor (depression) negatively influences the physiological health of individuals, resulting in an early onset of death. In a related study, individuals who were diagnosed with heart disease and who were depressed were significantly more likely to die sooner than were individuals with heart disease with no signs or diagnosis of depression (Glassman & Shapiro, 1998).

Shultz and colleagues (2000, 2005), Glassman and Shapiro (1998), and others are quick to note that they cannot establish through their research that depression definitively causes death. Rather, their research suggests one of two possible explanations for the correlations (see Chapter 2, Research Methods). One explanation, as noted previously, is that depression may influence the production of hormones such as epinephrine and other neurotransmitters that suppress the immune system. The suppressed system increases the risk of contracting viruses or other infectious diseases that can lead to mortality. A second possible explanation is that, due to depression, a person may engage in unhealthy behaviors that increase the probability of death. For example, a depressed individual may be more likely to use substances such as alcohol or illegal drugs to cope with the depression. Thus, behavioral factors such as substance abuse, initiated because of depression, could increase the risk of death.

Negative Emotions, Positive Effects Research on emotions and health show that it is also possible for negative emotions to have positive health consequences. In a review of the research on the health outcomes of negative affect, Mayne (1999) found that in some cases negative emotions can activate the sympathetic nervous system (SNS) and thereby stimulate the immune system. The ***sympathetic nervous system*** is part of the ***autonomic nervous system (ANS),*** or the part of our body that controls the automatic and involuntary functions that we do not think about but that are essential for living. For example, the ANS controls our heart rate, digestion, and perspiration. Another automatic or involuntary function is the body's physiological response to dangers, emergencies, or foreign organisms that invade the body. The sympathetic nervous system is responsible for mobilizing the body to respond to such dangers. This includes stimulating the immune system. Thus, negative affect, such as fear or fright, can stimulate the immune system to react to danger, possibly resulting in a positive outcome. We take a more in-depth look at the relationship between our emotions and our immune system in Chapter 8, Psychoneuroimmunology.

We noted that negative emotions can lead to behaviors that negatively affect health. Yet we find that negative emotions can also lead to health-enhancing behaviors. Studies suggest that negative emotions can increase the likelihood that individuals will seek timely medical help. Salovey, Rothman, Detweiler, and Steward (2000) and Mayne (1999) found that, when experiencing health problems, negative affect such as anxiety or depression may cause a person to perceive his or her physical condition more accurately and therefore increase the probability of that person seeking medical help. Consider this: An individual with a cold may become increasingly anxious if the cold lingers and produces thick mucus. That person's anxiety, a negative affect, may prompt him or her to seek medical care. In comparison, a person with a positive affect may not accurately assess the severity of the health condition or the fact that medical attention is needed. Someone with the same symptom—a lingering cold and thick mucus—who feels he or she can overcome the problem with sleep and copious amounts of liquids may not seek assistance. The lack of anxiety and the belief in his or her own skills may prevent that person from accurately assessing the severity of the health problem and from engaging in the appropriate health-seeking behavior.

Positive Emotions and Health If negative emotions can lead to poorer health outcomes, can positive emotions improve health status? We explore this question in depth in the following section on positive psychology. For now, however, it is important to note that some studies suggest such an association. For example, the role of ***positive affect*** on physiological health was demonstrated in a classic study by Cohen and colleagues (1991, 1995). In a laboratory-based study, these researchers exposed participants to a common cold virus to determine whether a person's affect influences disease progression. The study revealed that participants with a positive affect, here meaning positive feelings or emotions, at the time of exposure to the virus developed a less severe form of illness than did participants with a negative affect. Similarly, research by Moscowitz, Epel, and Acree (2008) found that positive affect can also decrease mortality rates among people with diabetes.

It might be tempting to conclude from the research that people who maintain a positive emotional demeanor will be less susceptible to severe illnesses. But keep in mind that affect is just one of a number of factors that influence health. An individual's physiological state, limitations, or dysfunctions will contribute also to the likelihood of contracting a disease, to the severity of the illness, and to its progression. In sum, current research shows that Hippocrates' initial premise was correct. Our positive and negative emotions do influence our well-being. He was incorrect, however, when characterizing the process by which emotions contribute to health.

PSYCHOLOGICAL FACTOR #2: HEALTH BEHAVIORS We reviewed a host of health behaviors in Chapter 5, Risky Health Behaviors, and discussed at length their positive and negative impacts on well-being. For example, we noted that although researchers have identified the benefits of consuming moderate amounts of red wine, excessive consumption or abuse of alcohol of any kind can have negative health consequences including gastrointestinal problems, heart disease, stroke, and cirrhosis of the liver (Centers for Disease Control, 2008; MMWR, 2004). We will not repeat the information from Chapter 5 in this section. But it is important to restate what we noted above: emotions can and often do influence health behaviors. For example, anxiety and depression are cited by some individuals as factors that contribute to their abuse of alcohol or other substances (Jessor, Donovan, & Costa, 1991). Thus, two psychological factors, health behaviors and emotions, can interact to influence health status.

SOCIOLOGICAL FACTOR #1: SOCIOECONOMIC CLASS AND INCOME In Chapter 3, Global Communicable and Chronic Disease, we identified the barriers to health care posed by lack of access to health insurance or to preventive medical care (Simon, Chan, & Forrest, 2008). What we did not state is that an individual's ***socioeconomic class (SEC)***—or the social and economic group that characterizes that person's social position in society—also greatly affects his or her access to care.

Socioeconomic class is a term developed by sociologists that categorizes individuals according to their positions in society as determined by their parents' level of education and occupation, their family's social status, and their family's income and wealth (Hout, Brooks, & Manzay, 1993; Liberatos, Link, & Kelsey, 1988). When evaluating the impact of socioeconomic class on health, researchers often use a simplified categorization scheme based primarily on household annual income levels: poor (less than $16,000), working class ($16,000 to $35,000), lower-middle class ($35,000 to $75,000), upper-middle class ($100,000 to $500,000), and wealthy (greater than $500,000) (Thompson & Hickey, 2005).

Without a doubt, SEC, defined here by household income, is a sociological factor that affects health by regulating access to medical care. The ability to pay for health insurance or to pay a medical provider's fee will influence a person's likelihood of seeking health care in a timely manner. Individuals unable to pay for needed health care due to limited income or lack of health insurance may delay seeking care, a decision that could aggravate the health problem. We explain the effect of socioeconomic status (income) on access to health care in greater detail in Chapter 12, Health Care Systems and Health Policy.

In addition to the inability to pay for care, studies suggest that people in lower socioeconomic groups may express negative affect more frequently than people in other SECs due largely to social environmental factors (Carroll, Smith, & Bennett, 2002). For example, lower SEC individuals are more likely to experience negative emotions, such as depression, which, as we mentioned already, can trigger illnesses or contribute to mortality (Gallo & Matthews, 2003). In addition, Cohen, Kaplan, and Salonen (1999) note that individuals in lower SEC groups (that is, poor or working poor) experience more stress (most often a negative affect) than those in higher SECs, a condition that can also lead to poorer well-being.

SOCIOLOGICAL FACTOR #2: FAMILY AND CULTURE Familial and cultural patterns of behavior, including diet and orientation to exercise and sports, also contribute to overall well-being. Take, for example, diet. Research on the nutritional practices of Japanese and Korean Americans reveals that many Asian diets minimize the risk of chronic diseases such as hypertension or digestive diseases (Park, Murphy, Sharmay, & Kolondel, 2005; Yang et al., 2007). Dietary practices in many Asian, specifically East Asian, countries include foods high in fiber, such as fruits, vegetables, and grain products, and low in fats.

Similarly, in a 20-year longitudinal study of deaths of middle-aged men due to chronic obstructive pulmonary disease (COPD; see Chapter 3, Global Communicable and Chronic Disease), researchers found that diets high in fruits and vitamin E decreased the incidences of death due to COPD among the cohort of Finnish, Italian, and Dutch men in the study (Walda et al., 2002). By contrast, as we also noted in Chapter 3, foods with high fat or high calorie content, such as pizza, cheeseburgers, and French fries—favorite American fast foods—are linked to chronic diseases, including heart diseases and diabetes (Scott, 2007; World Health Organization, 2002).

Nutrition and diet are important, but so is exercise. The International Association on the Study of Obesity reports that at least 30 minutes of exercise daily, together with a healthy diet, are required to reduce the risk of chronic diseases (Saris et al., 2003). Maintaining a regular exercise regimen is dependent on a number of factors, including past patterns and practices, which takes us back to the role of family or cultural determinants.

To summarize, the biopsychosocial model expands on the definition of health put forth in the biomedical model by including psychological, social, and emotional well-being as part of a holistic definition of health. Yet even with an expanded definition, researchers argue that the biopsychosocial model still places biology at the core of the definition. They contend that, rather than proposing a truly integrative model of health, the biopsychosocial model simply appends the psychological and sociological determinants of health as "add-ons" to the biomedical model (Armstrong, 2002). For this reason, we explore other models that offer alternative concepts of well-being that do not place biology at the center of the definition.

Wellness Model

The biopsychosocial model was the first to include psychological and social determinants as contributors to health outcomes. The ***wellness model*** includes the same psychological, social, and emotional factors included in the biopsychosocial model, but it adds two new dimensions: quality of life and spirituality.

QUALITY OF LIFE The wellness model defines health according to an individual's assessment of his or her own state of physical, mental, emotional, and spiritual well-being. For example, in a case study by Dinh and Groleau (2008), a Laotian man, Mr. B., summarizes his assessment of his overall well-being using quality of life and spirituality (see Box 6.1). In this study, Mr. B. unwillingly undergoes an emergency amputation of two fingers to protect him from a likely infection. According to the medical doctors on his case, the operation restored him to a state of good physical health. But, according to Mr. B., when surgeons removed his two fingers they also took part of his life and his life force. For Mr. B., the operation that Western medical doctors thought of as a lifesaving procedure diminished his ***quality of life*** and negatively affected his spiritual and overall well-being.

Similar examples of an individual's perception of wellness that departs from a biopsychosocial concept of health are found in the research literature on total knee replacement surgery, an increasingly common surgery for older adults in many Western cultures. Total knee replacement surgery usually is performed when a person's ***knee osteoarthritis,*** a form of arthritis in the knee that can become disabling over time, worsens to the point that surgery is required to relieve the pain or to correct a functional disability (see Chapter 10, Chronic Pain Management and Arthritis). Interestingly, research by Toye, Barlow, Wright, and Lamb (2006) shows that, for most patients, a decision to replace a dysfunctional knee is rarely explained by painful physical symptoms. Instead, Toye and colleagues (2006) found that a patient's feelings of vulnerability because of the unreliable knee, the desire not to depend on others for mobility, and the fatigue associated with an increased effort when performing daily tasks, in other words, quality of life issues, were the driving factors for knee replacement surgery. Thus Toye and colleagues (2006) suggest that decisions to have knee replacement surgery are based on the value placed on mobility, independence, and improved energy levels rather than on pain or discomfort. These concepts represent quality of life values that may not be considered important in a biomedical or biopsychosocial model of health but are essential factors in a wellness model.

BOX 6.1 Personal Meaning and Health: One Man's View of Wellness

Dinh and Groleau (2008) examine the case of a 49-year-old married Laotian man, Mr. B., living in Canada. According to their case study, Mr. B. was employed as an operator of heavy machinery at a factory in Canada. While at work, Mr. B. caught his glove in one of the heavy machines. The machine severed part of the third and fourth fingers on his left hand. He was immediately taken to the nearest hospital, where he waited approximately one hour before seeing a surgeon.

Mr. B. asked that his fingers be reattached, but the surgeon indicated that the tendons in his third and fourth fingers were dead and that the remaining parts of those fingers would have to be amputated. The surgeon's decision did not seem logical to Mr. B., who demonstrated that he could move the remaining segments of his fingers. The surgeon was not convinced, and three hours later, despite Mr. B.'s protests and pleas not to amputate, the medical staff prepped him for surgery to remove the remaining segments.

In the months after the surgery, Mr. B. received physical therapy to regain strength and movement in his hand. Doctors considered the surgery a success because it saved Mr. B. from probable infection of the hand and ensured that Mr. B. would return to an overall good state of health. Mr. B. did not share the doctor's point of view. Instead, he believed that the surgery "[took] his life."

According to Dinh and Groleau (2008), some Laotians believe that their health depends on the status of 12 souls that comprise a person's life force, known as *H'wen* (Dinh & Gorleau, 2008). The 12 souls correspond to parts of the body. The hands represent one of the souls. When Mr. B. lost his fingers, he lost one of his life forces. Thus in this case study, Mr. B.'s health, according to the wellness model, was significantly impaired on two fronts: psychosocial and spiritual. First, unable to resume work as a heavy machinery operator, Mr. B. was unable to earn a living and provide for his family. His quality of life was affected by his inability to assume his role as the principal wage earner in the family. Second, the loss of his fingers represented a lost energy force and resulted in diminished spiritual well-being.

When explaining his feelings in French, Mr. B could only say he felt "*triste*," or sad. But, when talking with Laotian friends, his wife, or others who understood the Laotian culture, he explained that he felt indignation and felt unworthy of respect.

Mr. B.'s inability to return to his job affected his sense of responsibility and obligation to his family. His feelings of indignation and of being unworthy of respect reflect the influence of Laotian culture. It suggests a social influence that impacts his emotional state of health and a spiritual influence consistent with his Buddhist beliefs. Mr. B.'s case demonstrates how spirituality, quality of life, culture, and emotional health all contribute to his assessment of his overall well-being. Not surprisingly, he currently views his overall quality of life as poor.

SPIRITUALITY The wellness model also addresses spiritual health, faith, and religion—topics that are not usually included in psychological research. Some scientists consider ***spirituality*** a pseudoscience or a primitive superstition and therefore not something to be included in rigorous studies that explain individual health outcomes. Recently, however, more researchers have examined the relationship between spirituality and health (see Chapter 7, Stress and Coping). The new research suggests a change among current scientists, at least those in the health fields, who believe that spirituality is essential for some individuals to obtain optimal health (Diaz, 1993; Myslakidou et al., 2008; Seaward, 1991).

By spirituality, researchers are not necessarily referring to religious dogma. Rather, studies focus on the impact of an individual's philosophy, values, and meaning of life (Mullen, McDermott, Gold, & Belcastro, 1996) on health status. Scientists suggest that spirituality may afford individuals peace and tranquility in the face of stressful events and a sense of meaningfulness that provides them with direction and fulfillment

(Perrin & McDermott, 1997). In addition, some spiritual practices promote healthy behaviors. For example, the dietary practices of Muslims and some Christian denominations include abstinence from alcohol; this can be a health-enhancing behavior, particularly for those who otherwise would be inclined to consume alcohol in excess (see Chapter 5, Risky Health Behaviors).

Recent studies examining the relationship between spirituality and well-being among migraine suffers provide additional support for the health-enhancing effects of spirituality. ***Migraines*** are considered a neurological disorder of unknown origins. The symptoms generally include painful headaches that do not respond to over-the-counter pain medications, nausea, and vomiting. Researchers believe that migraines may be associated with depression and anxiety, suggesting an emotional basis for the illness.

One recent study explored the effects of four types of meditation techniques—spiritual meditation, internally focused meditation, externally focused meditation, and muscle relaxation—on migraine suffers to determine which, if any, resulted in significantly improved outcomes (Wachholtz & Pargament, 2008). Each of the 83 study participants in the migraine study learned and practiced one of the four techniques for 20 minutes a day for a total of 30 days. The results of pre-post test measures (see Chapter 2, Research Methods) revealed that participants who used the spiritual meditation techniques fared much better than those using any of the other three approaches. The spiritual meditation users reported a decrease in frequency of headaches and in negative affect. In addition, they reported an increase in pain tolerance, self-efficacy, and overall wellbeing (Wachholtz & Pargament, 2008).

In sum, this particular study and other on the effects of spirituality on well-being suggests that spirituality offers some individuals tranquility in troubled times, guidance on healthy lifestyles and behaviors, emotional wellness, and an ability to regulate pain levels, all of which contribute to well-being.

We need to make one additional point about the role of spirituality. Individuals incorporate spiritual practices into their healing traditions even in cultures in which the biomedical model of health is strongly favored. The study with migraine sufferers is one example. Consider also the case presented in Box 6.2. Dr. Paul Farmer, a physician, was reminded that, even in Western cultures, individuals combine spirituality with medical science in their efforts to overcome illnesses.

BOX 6.2 Medicine and Spirituality: A Compatible Combination in Western Medicine?

Dr. Paul Farmer is not your "average" doctor. Raised on a boat and in a bus during his childhood, Dr. Farmer's early years accurately could be called atypical. Perhaps his early experience living in nontraditional environments led him to a career caring for the poorest of the poor in Haiti, Peru, Cuba, and Russia (see Figure 6.3).

Dr. Farmer is an infectious disease specialist, someone who studies and treats contagious diseases. Given his special interests, it is not surprising that Dr. Farmer would travel to developing countries (see Chapter 3, Global Communicable and Chronic Disease) in which infectious diseases are quite common. But it was during his work in Haiti that he was reminded of the dual presence of medical science and spirituality in Haitian and Western cultures.

One year, while treating patients in Haiti for tuberculosis (TB; see Chapter 3, Global Communicable and Chronic Diseases), Dr. Farmer designed a study to test an idea debated by his health care staff. He wanted to understand whether the poor health outcomes of impoverished patients like those in Haiti could be attributed to economic conditions and the inability to pay for care or whether their outcomes were rooted

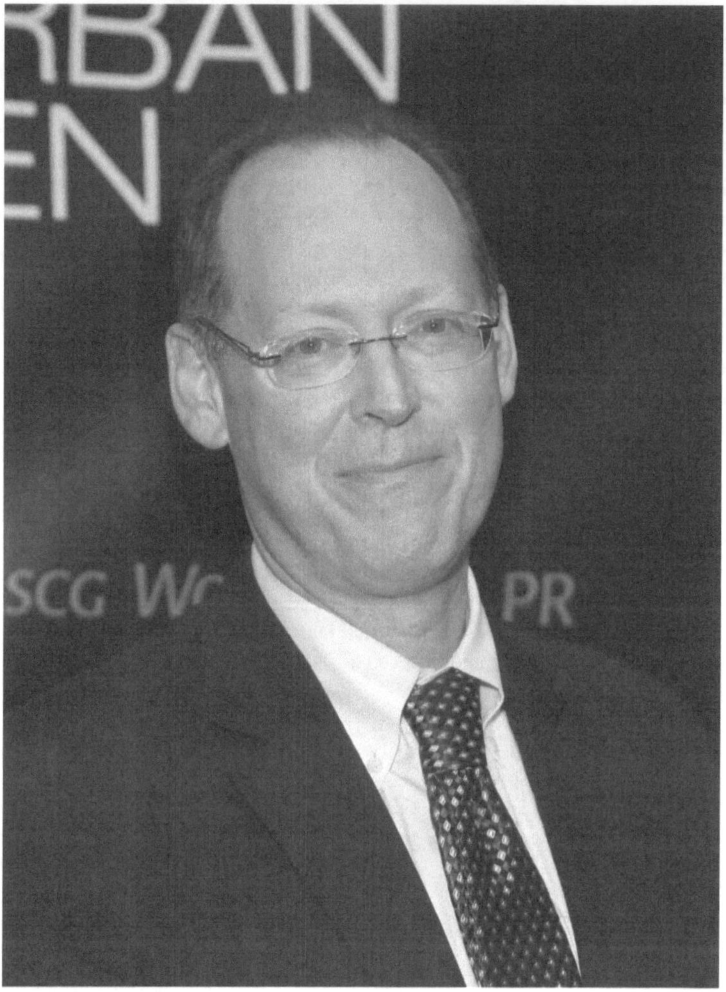

FIGURE 6.3 Dr. Paul Farmer.

Source: UNICEF (2008)/ Getty #125693681

in their belief that illnesses had spiritual origins. In Haiti, some individuals believe that Illnesses are sent by enemies through sorcery (Kidder, 2003). Dr. Farmer's staff proposed that individuals who believed that illnesses were curses sent by others would be less likely to follow the medical regimen to treat their TB.

To test the idea, Dr. Farmer divided his TB patients into two groups. The medication-only group would receive the necessary treatment for TB, but the medication plus services group would receive the medicine in addition to regular visits from community health workers and cash stipends for child care and for travel by public transport to the nearest village. Dr. Farmer interviewed all of his patients at the beginning of the study and again one year later. Farmer found that few patients in either group admitted believing that TB was sent to them from an enemy via sorcery. In spite of their denials, Dr. Farmer's results suggested otherwise. One year after beginning the study, less than half (48%) of the medication-only group was cured of TB. By comparison, all of the medication-plus-extra-services patients had fully recovered (Kidder, 2003).

As part of the one-year follow-up, Dr. Farmer asked his patients their views on the origins of their disease. He revisited one woman in the medication-plus-services group who, the previous year, seemed offended at his question about her beliefs in the origin of diseases. At the time, she stated that she knew that TB came from "people coughing germs" (Kidder, 2003, p. 35). But one year later, the same woman, now fully recovered from TB, admitted that she knew who sent her the sickness. She vowed revenge on the person.

Realizing that the woman was admitting that she believed in sorcery as a source of the disease, Dr. Farmer asked why she used the medicine to combat TB. The woman's response illustrates the duality of medical science and spirituality in Haiti and, ironically, in the United States. In Haitian Creole, she responded, "*Cheri ... eske-w pa ka kom prann bagay ki pa senp?*" (Kidder, 2003, p. 35). Translated, the woman asked Dr. Farmer, "Honey, are you incapable of complexity?"

The woman's question reminded Dr. Farmer of himself and others he knew in the United States who held similar complex views on faith and medicine. In fact, there are many examples of such complexities in Western medicine. Chapels in hospitals and chaplains in medical centers are but two examples of the complex relationship between faith and health in modern cultures. Many individuals who seek treatment from health care providers in hospitals also call on their faith, an act that demonstrates their values and belief structures, to guide medical staff and to speed healing and recovery.

From the research, it is clear that spirituality plays a health-enhancing role for many individuals and in many cultures. We will see later that spirituality is also recognized as a central component of well-being in cultures that practice traditional forms of medicine.

Social Ecological Model

The biopsychosocial model proposes that biological, psychological and social factors contribute to overall well-being. The wellness model includes two additional dimensions: spiritual health and perceived quality of life as essential to overall well-being. Because we have explored the biological, psychological, emotional, and social environmental determinants of health in the previous models, here we focus on three determinants unique to the ***social ecological model***: physical and psychological environments, health systems, and health policy.

ENVIRONMENTAL DETERMINANTS The ***ecological model*** identifies two types of environments. First is a social environment, similar to that proposed in the biopsychosocial model, that includes the interpersonal, familial, and cultural factors that affect an individual's emotional state of well-being. The second environment is a physical space and the perceived quality of that space (see again Figure 1.3 in Chapter 1, An Interdisciplinary View of Health).

Physical Environmental Determinants When exploring environmental influences on health in Chapter 3, Global, Communicable and Chronic Disease, and Chapter 4, Theories and Models of Health Behavior Change, we discussed the effects of contaminated environments on overall well-being. We noted that hazards such as toxic waste sites contribute to high incidences of diseases and high infant mortality rates, especially among the poor and working classes. Specifically, we noted that cancers and severe respiratory illnesses have been linked to these sites, which are a physical environmental determinant of ill health.

The effect of the environment on health outcomes is not a new discovery. Sir Edwin Chadwick, an early proponent of the association between environment and health, demonstrated the dangerous consequences of some environments on individual health in England in the mid-1800s. Sir Chadwick's research, summarized in Box 6.3, documented the health consequences of individuals living and working in unsanitary conditions in urban and rural England. In addition, Chadwick showed that disparities in environmental conditions are correlated with socioeconomic status. He demonstrated that the lower socioeconomic classes, specifically the poor and working classes, were more likely to be exposed to health-compromising environmental conditions in their neighborhoods as well as their workplace environments, than were individuals in the higher socioeconomic classes. Unfortunately, health compromised living and working environments for people in the lower SECs are present in most countries even today (Northridge & Sclar, 2003; Schultz & Northridge, 2004; Schultz, Williams, Israel, & Lempert, 2002).

The ecological model, in conjunction with Chadwick's work, identifies the hazardous effects of some physical environments on well-being. In England in the 1800s, many neighborhoods were without sewer or drainage systems. The lack of adequate waste disposal systems (an environmental determinant) resulted in polluted water systems and soiled streets, footpaths and grounds. Waste disposal systems are usually the purview of municipal or regional governments and are indicative of the health policies of that region. But, it is also important to point out that in this case, the water systems were contaminated by waste products generated by individuals and businesses. Thus, individuals also contributed to the environmental hazard.

Health Systems and Health Policy Another unique aspect of the social ecological model is its inclusion of health systems and health policy, specifically the agencies and regulations respectively that define the structure of health care and that regulate its services. Both are included as distinct determinants of health outcomes.

Thomas Southward Smith found that the absence of sewers and drainage systems in England in the 1830s and 1840s, a health policy decision, was correlated with the frequency of high fevers among residents. Smith's finding is consistent with Chadwick's work, which also attests to the relationship between the physical environmental conditions in poor neighborhoods and the poor health outcomes of its inhabitants. Both Chadwick and Smith understood that health policy initiatives could influence health status and could either enhance or impair the health outcomes of poorer citizens. Their work supports the role of policy as a determinant of health (Gee & Payne-Sturges, 2004).

Consider a more current example. In the United States, policy decisions by local or regional governments may result in a solid waste treatment plant being built in or near a residential district. In many instances, such facilities are built in neighborhoods in which the majority of the residents either are members of minority groups or belong to the poor or working classes (CERD Working Group on Health & Environmental Health, 2008). Residents in such neighborhoods understand that a waste treatment plant could produce unpleasant odors and discharges that could also cause or aggravate respiratory health problems. If, as a result of the new treatment plant, some residents developed respiratory illnesses, it would be incorrect to assume that the residents' own health behaviors caused the illness. Rather, it is equally as likely that the policy decision to locate a waste treatment plant in a specific neighborhood created the conditions that triggered the respiratory health problems of residents.

Psychological Environment and Health Environment can also be defined as the quality of an individual's physical space as determined by psychosocial variables. For example, overcrowded neighborhoods or communities with high crime rates are psychosocial variables that influence the quality of life and overall well-being.

BOX 6.3 Environment, Socioeconomic Class, and Health

In 1847, Thomas Southwood Smith observed that there was an interesting relationship between the location of sewers on a city map in London and the outbreak of fevers in the same city (Hamlin & Sheard, 1998). He found what we would probably call a significant correlation between the fevers—an individual or biological determinant of health—and the existence of sewers, an environmental health determinant, which is regulated by health policy decisions.

Smith's observation explained what we now clearly know about the association between unsanitary environmental conditions and health. However, in the early- to mid-1800s, this argument met with sharp resistance.

Sir Edwin Chadwick, a devout public health advocate, encountered similar resistance when he observed a related phenomenon. Concerned about the living conditions of the working class and the effects of these conditions on their health, Sir Edwin lobbied the English legislative bodies to examine the public health conditions of the poor and working classes in England. In 1832, England was preparing to revisit the Poor Laws, a set of laws designed to provide equitable assistance to the poor to help improve their standard of living. Chadwick was convinced, however, that no significant improvements could be made unless one also addressed the health status and living conditions of the working class.

To this end, Chadwick conducted a survey of adult and infant death rates of the three principal classes in Great Britain in the mid-1800s: the gentry (landowner and aristocrats or professionals), tradesmen (shopkeepers), and finally the wage-earning working class. He summarized his findings in a report entitled *Report from the Poor Law Commissions on an Inquiry into the Sanitary Conditions of the Labouring [Working] Population of Great Britain* (Chadwick, 1842). Two important statistics included in the survey were a comparison of the mortality rates for adults in three socioeconomic classes and infant death rates among these same three classes, as shown below.

Adult Mortality and Infant Death Rates, England, 1842

	Mean Age of Death		*Infant Deaths*
Class	*Urban (London)*	*Rural (Countryside)*	*Per 1,000 Births*
Gentry/professional	44 years	35 years	100 deaths
Tradesmen/shopkeepers	23 years	22 years	167 deaths
Wage/working class	22 years	15 years	250 deaths

The statistics supported Chadwick's hypothesis: The living and working conditions of the three classes explained much of the disparity in mortality statistics. The English wage and working classes in the 1840s could expect, on average, to live only half as long as individuals in the gentry class. In addition, babies born to parents in the laboring classes were 2.5 times more likely to die before age five than were infants born to parents in the gentry or aristocratic classes.

Chadwick argued that the wage-earning and laboring classes lived in the most unsanitary conditions and were exposed to the harshest work environments. He believed that these conditions directly contributed to unusually high early-adult mortality and high infant mortality rates.

Using these statistics, Sir Edwin convinced the English legislature to pass the Public Health Act and Nuisance Removal and Disease Prevention Act of 1848. Unsatisfied with the weak content of the act, Chadwick continued to advocate for better health conditions for the laboring class.

In Chapter 5, Risky Health Behaviors, we explained how a neighborhood's high crime rate can affect one's health even if an individual is not, him or herself, a victim. For example, people who perceive that their neighborhood is less safe due to crime will be less likely to engage in outdoor exercise in their community. Limited access to exercise will have a direct impact on well-being.

There is another way in which high crime rates can affect emotional health. Consider this: Residents in high-crime neighborhoods may be more anxious about leaving or returning home at night and more apt to listen for threatening sounds from the street while at home. Increased anxiety or greater emotional distress about one's safety or the safety of one's family, even when "safely" at home, may have long-term consequences for well-being. We briefly described the effects of stress on well-being in the previous section and explore the issue more fully in Chapter 7, Stress and Coping.

Workplace Environments as Determinants of Emotional Health Overcrowding and crime are tangible environmental factors that affect psychological health. Yet psychological factors in the environment that also impact health outcomes can be subtle. One example is the effect of the workplace on individuals' physiological or emotional health. Kawano (2008) conducted a study among nurses in Japan to determine whether working in specific medical services units, such as the operating room, intensive care units, and surgical or internal medicine units, caused higher levels of emotional distress or physical fatigue among the nurses. The results showed that, in fact, nurses in each of the three special units experienced higher levels of emotional distress than their colleges in nonspeciality units. Nurses working in operating rooms reported higher levels of fatigue, whereas their colleagues in the intensive care units (units that care for patients with critical medical needs) reported higher levels of anxiety. Finally, nurses in surgical or internal medicine units reported higher levels of depression.

These are interesting results, to be sure. But why should one type of medical service cause more fatigue or emotional stress than another? The answer may be clear when we consider what is at stake. The work performed by nurses is vital to returning a patient to a state of overall well-being. In settings like the operating room or in critical care units, unintentional mistakes can seriously impair a patient's health or even contribute to death, a weighty responsibility for any caregiver. Perhaps, then, nurses' higher levels of anxiety or depression reflect their concern about the consequences of an error, the potential for loss of life, and the likely emotional cost borne by them if they were responsible for a mistake resulting in the death of a patient.

Summary

To review, the definition of health has evolved over the past several centuries. The discovery of microorganisms and their role in causing illnesses led Western scientists to focus on the physiological or biological causes of illness and to define health as the absence of disease, as represented by the biomedical view of health. Now new definitions have led to a shift from the biomedical perspective to a more holistic view of health similar to that espoused by earlier cultures.

Health psychologists, medical sociologists, and public health experts currently argue for a broader definition of health, best conceptualized as overall well-being. The biopsychosocial model was one of the first models to expand the definition of health by adding social and psychological factors to the concept of well-being. The wellness model contributed a spiritual dimension to well-being and redefined wellness as an individual's own assessment of their status, whereas the social ecological model adds the physical environmental determinants as well as the role of health systems and health policy on individual health outcomes.

In sum, concepts of health and well-being have shifted over time, beginning with the concept of well-being as a mind–body connection, moving to a physiologically based determinant of health, only to return once again to a view of health as a holistic or ecological concept. Still, some health psychologists contend that the definition of well-being is incomplete. Some advocate for a need to examine the positive as well as the negative aspects of well-being in order to provide a balanced perspective of wellness.

SECTION II. POSITIVE PSYCHOLOGY

Positive psychology seems like an odd-sounding "pop psychology" name for a theory. As such, it may be tempting to dismiss the concept as trendy. But, as you will see, it is neither new nor trendy. Positive psychology builds on the wellness model of health and is, according to Seligman (2002), a more complete and balanced perspective of the human experience (Seligman, Steen, Park, & Peterson, 2000). Specifically, positive psychology involves a systematic study of the factors that enhance and maintain an individual's state of well-being.

BOX 6.4 Seligman's Classification of Character Strengths

Seligman suggests that individuals who strive to achieve six universal virtues, here meaning virtues found in many cultures, religions, and philosophical traditions, and 24 strengths will live a more fulfilled and happy life. The positive effects that result from a happier and more fulfilled life will lead to a greater likelihood of positive, healthy outcomes and overall well-being.

In essence, for Seligman, positive psychology returns the field of psychology to its mission, which is to make normal people's lives more fulfilling and productive (Clay, 1977). His work seeks to understand the factors that contribute to such an outcome. Thus, positive psychology moves away from the biomedical concept of health, which focuses on identifying, isolating, and repairing problems, to a more holistic or ecological perspective regarding human potentials, motives, and capacities but one that explains the positive and negative contributions to overall well-being (Seligman & Csikszentmihalyi, 2000; Sheldon & King, 2001).

Defining Positive Psychology

Martin Seligman and Mihaly Csikszentmihalyi (2000) pioneered the concept of positive psychology. In their view, much of psychology over the past 60 years focused on issues of mental illness, damage, or dysfunction (Seligman, 2002). According to some, Seligman suggests that psychology's focus on mental illness positioned it as a science of pathology and weakness rather than a science of health, well-being, and strength (Held, 2005).

Consequently, Seligman and Csikszentmihalyi (2000) proposed to correct what they characterized as an imbalance in the field by identifying and explaining the factors that lead to overall wellbeing, thriving communities, and satisfied individuals and families (Seligman & Csikszentmihalyi, 2000). Seligman, Park, and Peterson (2004) and later Peterson and Seligman (2004) proposed that six "virtues," along with 24 signature character strengths (See Box 6.4) that represent positive traits, contribute to life satisfaction and a more meaningful life (Park, Peterson, & Seligman, 2004). The five character strengths most strongly associated with life satisfaction are presented in Table 6.1.

Positive versus Negative Psychology?

For some, the term *positive psychology* implies that there is also a "negative psychology." Most likely Seligman's characterization of some fields as "negative social science and psychology" created the dichotomy that fueled the debate (Held, 2005). Indeed, few would choose to be associated with a discipline within psychology, or any field for that matter, that is characterized as "negative." Although Seligman later rephrased his criticism of other disciplines of psychology in terms that are less stigmatizing, the comparison between positive psychology and other areas within the field continues to cause conflicts about the role and relative contribution of—even the need for—positive psychology as its own discipline.

It would be easy to become enmeshed in a war of words in the characterization of some areas of psychology as positive or negative. But to do so would miss the principal intent of positive psychology, which is to seek and discover an optimal balance between "positive" and "negative" thinking (Seligman, 2002) and to understand psychological phenomena in their totality (Carstensen & Charles, 2003). In

TABLE 6.1 Five Character Strengths Most Strongly Correlated with Life Satisfaction

Strength	*Description*
Hope	[Optimism, future-mindedness, future orientation]: Expecting the best in the future and working to achieve it; believing that a good future is something that can be brought about
Zest	[Vitality, enthusiasm, vigor, energy]: Approaching life with excitement and energy; not doing things halfway or halfheartedly, living life as an adventure; feeling alive and activated
Gratitude	Being aware of and thankful for the good things that happen; taking time to express thanks
Curiosity	[Interest, novelty-seeking, openness to experiences]: Taking an interest in all ongoing experiences; finding all subjects and topics fascinating; exploring and discovering
Love	Valuing close relationships with others, in particular those in which sharing and caring are reciprocated; being close to people

Source: Strengths of character & well-being. Journal of Social and Clinical Psychology, 23(5), 603–619. Park, N., Peterson, C., & Seligman, M. E. P. (2004).

other words, positive and negative influences contribute to the outcomes, states, emotions, and health of individuals. To understand an individual's end state, we need to examine both.

Positive Psychology and Health

After more than 60 years of research using a "disease" model approach to health, Seligman contends that we really are no better at actually preventing negative psychological outcomes or damage than we were when the research began. Rather, he contends that the most effective way to prevent illnesses is to focus on the positive goals of building competencies and on the reinforcing factors that prevent negative events from occurring (Seligman & Csikszentmihalyi, 2000). In this way, positive psychology may be of particular importance to the field of health psychology because it may facilitate a transition from the biopsychosocial to the social ecological approach by examining the multiple contributions, both positive and negative, to well-being.

What are the factors that help build healthier, satisfied, thriving individuals and communities? According to current studies, personal traits such as an individual's subjective sense of well-being, optimism, happiness, self-determination, and positive emotional states contribute to a positive psychology and well-being (Diener, 2000; Myers, 2000; Ryan & Deci, 2000; Salovey, Rothman, Detweiler, & Steward, 2000; Taylor et al., 2000). Like all individuals, thriving and happy people exist in a social context that includes other people, places, and institutions. Therefore, positive psychological states are influenced also by social and environmental factors that include interpersonal relationships, social networks (Cohen, 2004; Ray, 2004; Taylor & Turner, 2001), religion and religious faith (Myers, 2000), and external factors, including socioeconomic status (Coburn, 2004; Wilkinson, 1996).

How do we know that positive psychological states also contribute to our well-being? Consider for a moment the research on ***optimism,*** here meaning the view that situations and events will work out for the best, however *best* is defined. Studies on the effect of optimism among cancer patients, for example, have found an association between optimism and better psychological and social adjustment to their illness (Lechner et al., 2006). Researchers have also found that patients who reported higher levels of optimism also reported lower levels of depression or anxiety about the illness (Bjorck, Hopp, & Jones, 1999; Schnoll, Knowles, & Harlow, 2002). What is more, some cancer patients with an optimistic perspective also believe that they can influence their situation and thereby achieve a better outcome (Folkman & Greer, 2002). If optimism has a direct effect on emotional health, and if positive emotional health can directly influence our physiological states, then we may be correct in concluding that positive psychological perspectives indirectly enhance health.

Work by Taylor and colleagues (2000) also demonstrates the positive effects of optimism on indirect health factors that affect well-being. For example, Taylor et al. (2000) found that optimistic, self-confident people have more social support, here meaning assistance and help from friends, family, or work associates. As we will see in Chapter 7, Stress and Coping, social networks buffer individuals from the effects of negative or stressful situations and enhance their ability to cope with the challenges. Because, as noted earlier, stress can have detrimental physical and emotional effects, factors that minimize stress will enhance health outcomes.

Other studies in the field of behavioral medicine also demonstrate the health benefits obtained from a positive, optimistic state. Ironson and Hayward (2008) and Ironson, Stuetzle, and Fletcher (2006) suggest that optimism, together with active coping strategies and spirituality, predict a slower progression of HIV disease in HIV-positive individuals. A slower progression of HIV may delay the onset of symptoms associated with the illness as well as slow the debilitating effects of the disease itself.

The main point of positive psychology is that we understand only part of our human nature if we focus exclusively on pathology, disorder, or dysfunction. To understand the full human experience and how to make people's lives more fulfilling and satisfying, we need to study the "normal," positive, and productive state of human functioning as well as the disordered or damaged states. As we will see in the following section, for followers of traditional, complementary or alternative medicine an understanding of the positive or normal state is also integral to their health beliefs and practices.

Critiques of Positive Psychology

In principle, positive psychology aims to present a more balanced view of the factors that affect outcomes. There are, however, criticisms of the concept. Two issues in particular, the "happiness" approach and the universality of the concept, appear to be the most frequently cited limitations of the positive psychology movement.

HAPPINESS PSYCHOLOGY Remember our earlier caution of not becoming embroiled in a war of words? Some researchers argue that the principal focus of positive psychology is to study what makes people happy. When stated in this fashion, positive psychology seems insubstantial. Yet recent research by Perez-Alvarez (2016) and earlier work by Held (2002) suggest that this critique involves more than just a war a words. They question whether there are more important values than striving for happiness (Perez-Alvarez, 2016). Held (2002) goes further by questioning whether a positive attitude is really necessary to achieve an overall sense of well-being. He asks whether accentuating the positive and eliminating the negative is really beneficial for one's overall physical and mental health. These questions appear to address core components of the theory that must be addressed.

When, however, looking more broadly, the concept of "happiness" also includes research to understand gratitude, forgiveness, awe, inspiration, hope, curiosity, and laughter (Gable & Haidt, 2005). The work of the Truth and Reconciliation Commission in South Africa is one recent example of an application of positive psychology in its broadest definition (see Box 6.5 and Figure 6.4).

Widely acclaimed as one of the factors that aided South Africa's peaceful transition and positive development in the aftermath of apartheid, the Truth and Reconciliation Commission's approach to conflict resolution and healing has been praised and emulated around the world (Philpott, 2009). More importantly, it was integral to forging a new relationship among ethnic groups that would allow the citizens of South Africa to forgive the atrocities of the past and inspire them to work toward building a stronger and more unified country.

If positive psychology is defined simply as what makes people happy, it would seem to have limited application to the work in health psychology. The broader implications of "happiness," as seen through the research and work on forgiveness, would support a central role for this field, one that contributes to our understanding of health-enhancing behaviors.

UNIVERSALITY OF POSITIVE PSYCHOLOGY A more compelling criticism of the field is that the new discipline may not be applicable to some people or cultures in spite of its claims of being a universal phenomenon (Aspinwall & Staudinger, 2003). As Diener and Suh (2000) note, in North American cultures there is a strong psychological pressure to be happy. In fact, Diener and Suh characterize it as an inviolable individual right, particularly in cultures with strong beliefs in individualism and self-determination. Critics argue that if, as in some cultures, there is no universal belief in the right of individual happiness then, by definition, positive psychology may not be universal.

BOX 6.5 The South African Truth and Reconciliation Commission: Forgiveness in Post-Apartheid South Africa

The full scope of the atrocities committed under the apartheid government in South Africa may never be known. ***Apartheid,*** a social and political policy of racial segregation enforced by the government of South Africa, was finally dismantled in 1992, but not before thousands of South Africans were killed or severely tortured to protect the apartheid system.

Following decades of forced segregation, forced removals from homes and communities, and restrictions on employment and even on education, South Africa's black, colored, and Indian citizens finally won the opportunity to live without the imposition of socially unjust rules instituted under apartheid. As they embarked on the job of forming a new, democratic government, the country faced the daunting task of healing a nation riddled for decades with the racial animus caused by the apartheid system. Central to that task was finding a way to help foster forgiveness between the races.

South Africa's Truth and Reconciliation Commission was charged with the responsibility of discovering the truth about the thousands of atrocities committed during apartheid while simultaneously moving the country forward in peace. Archbishop Desmond Tutu, the first black Anglican archbishop in South Africa, headed the commission (see Figure 6.4). With his leadership, the commission pioneered a model by which perpetrators of violence and torture could face their victims and their families. By truthfully confessing their crimes, the guilty could seek forgiveness from their victims, and family members of victims could learn the truth about the brutal torture or murder of their loved ones, again from the confessions of the perpetrators of the acts. The act of public confession and contrition was seen as one way to begin the healing process that could allow South Africa's diverse racial groups to survive and to thrive as a nation (Gobodo-Madikizela, 2002, 2003). It was one way to begin to repair the emotional and psychological damage experienced by the nation.

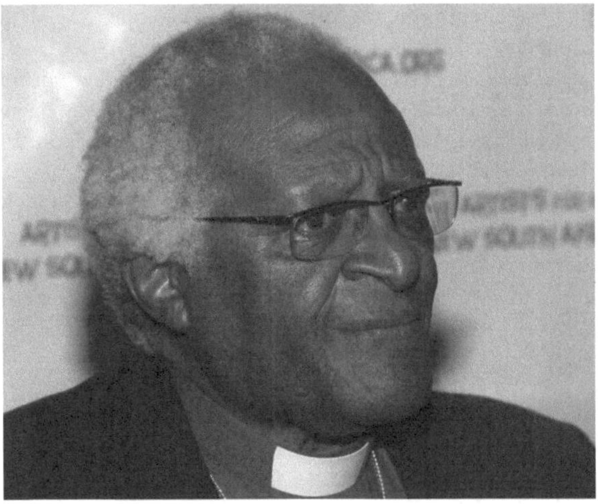

FIGURE 6.4 **Archbishop Desmond Tutu.** Chair of South Africa's Truth and Reconciliation Commission, Archbishop Tutu helped guide South Africans through a post-apartheid healing process.

Source: Paul Chiasson/Associated Press

The applicability of positive psychology is also challenged when concepts that are interpreted as positive or that elicit positive connotations in one culture have both negative and positive meanings in another. Take, for example, the concept of "sympathy." In Western cultures, sympathy is a positive emotion suggesting the ability to understand another's position. It is one of several strengths that lead to the six virtues identified by Seligman. In Chinese culture, sympathy also has a distinctly negative connotation, meaning to commiserate with or to have sympathy with someone's misfortune (Sundararajan, 2005). Thus, a positive concept in one culture can be linked to both positive or negative concepts in another. The point here is that the notion that positive characteristics are universally seen as positive in all cultures can be easily challenged by examining the understood meaning of words across cultures.

What is more, Confucianism, an Eastern philosophy that emphasizes human morality and moral development of the individual, proposes that negative emotions play an important role in the development of virtue, the underpinnings of happiness and well-being, according to Seligman (Sundararajan, 2005). In other words, Eastern philosophy holds that negative emotions are critical for the full development of the individual. In defense, positive psychology does not deny the existence of negative emotions. But it appears that it fails to consider negative emotional development as integral to positive emotions and outcomes.

We close this section with one additional observation. Recently, researchers have re-examined the role of ***pessimism*** as an adaptive, and hence positive, approach to select issues or problems. In fact, some contend that pessimism may work to promote problem solving (Aspinwall & Staudinger, 2003). They note specifically that ***defensive pessimism,*** a coping strategy that keeps disappointments and expectations in check (Norem, 2001), may be adaptive when responding to negative outcomes.

Defensive pessimism may be a particularly advantageous emotion for disenfranchised groups in societies. For such groups, defensive pessimism may help, albeit nominally, to cope with frequent encounters of disappointments and rejections caused, in part, by that group's status in society. For example, minority groups that experience discrimination based on their ethnicity may employ defensive pessimism when involved in social or work settings in the majority culture to minimize the adverse effects of exclusion or other forms of rejection. Therefore, although Seligman believes that pessimism is maladaptive (Held, 2005), for some it may be an effective method of coping with a myriad of negative social environmental issues that affect emotional well-being.

Does positive psychology contribute to our understanding of emotional health? It would seem so, in spite of its limitations. No single model or theory will contain all the elements needed to explain behaviors or outcomes. As we indicated in Chapter 4, Theories and Models of Health Behavior Change, models often borrow concepts to build stronger models. Positive psychology could be an important contribution to existing theories, reminding us that to understand the full spectrum of human behavior we need to identify all determinants that impact well-being.

SECTION III. TRADITIONAL MEDICINES

Models of health developed by Western societies have identified biology, sociology, psychology, emotion, environments, and health systems and policy as integral to individual well-being. These same factors have also been identified and used in traditional medicines.

Traditional medicine is a term that refers to medical practices, knowledge, and beliefs in cultures whose practices predate those of Western medicine. It includes the use of plant-, animal-, and mineral-based medicines, as well as spiritual techniques to administer to an individual's health needs (World Health Organization, 2003).

Most traditional medicines share four core principles: a belief in a connection among the individual, Earth, and a life or energy force; a belief that a person's state of health reflects a balance or harmony of three connected elements—the individual, Earth, and the energy force; a belief that treatment for a health problem involves the whole individual—physical, emotional or mental, and spiritual; and a belief in the use of herbal remedies or other practices such as ritual chants, acupuncture, bone setting, or smudging (that is, using smoke from burning herbs to cleanse negative energies around a person) (Broome & Broome, 2007; Lam, 2001).

In some countries, such as China, Korea, Ghana, and South Africa, traditional and Western medicine approaches are not only widely available, they are often used together to address individual health needs. For example, the South African government integrated the ***sangomas***, indigenous healers used by many rural South Africans, into the nation's health care system (Africa First, 2008; International on Line, 2004; World Health Organization, 2003). Now, South Africans can choose to receive care from either a Western-trained medical doctor or a *sangoma* and have the cost of care paid for or supplemented by the nation's health care system.

It is important to state that the integration of traditional and Western health practices, as in the case of South Africa, only formalizes a long-standing practice of consulting both Western and traditional medicines. Remember Angelita from our opening story? She consulted a modern health professional but also accepted the assistance of a *curandero,* one type of traditional healer. One reason people use both health approaches is that they believe that each addresses different health needs. Thus they seek to maximize the advantages and minimize the disadvantages of each technique. Interestingly, even some health care providers report consulting both Western medicine and traditional healers for their own health care needs (Bucko & Cloud, 2008; Hon et al., 2005; Lam, 2001; Wong et al., 2006).

Contributions of Traditional Medicine

Would it surprise you to learn that approximately 25% of all Western medicines are made from plants used first by traditional healers (World Health Organization, 2003)? This little-known fact is actually taught to children, although they may not be aware of the message at the time. Consider, for example, the Walt Disney movie *Pocahontas*. Pocahontas, the daughter of the chief of the Powhatan nation, gives John Smith, an English settler, ground bark from a willow tree to ease his pain from a gunshot wound. The bark contains ***salicylic acid,*** an ingredient that controls pain and reduces fever (University of Arkansas, Division of Agriculture, 2007). Pharmaceutical companies, the manufacturers of modern medicines, have developed a chemical equivalent of ground willow bark to relieve similar aches and pain. We call it ***aspirin***. Scientists learned to chemically reproduce the same ingredients found in the willow tree used by Native Americans and to mass produce it for general use.

Today, scientists continue to copy and reproduce for mass distribution the medicinal elements found in plants. Take, for example, the plant ***hoodia gordonii***. "Hoodia," as it is known in the United States, is a natural plant found in southern Africa used for centuries by the ***Sans*** people, a nomadic group living in the Kalahari desert of southern Africa. The *Sans* use hoodia gordonii to suppress appetite. You may wonder why a nomadic group would want to suppress their appetites. Simply put, the *Sans* hunt for their food. A hunt for a wildebeest or eland large enough for the needs of the tribe may take several days and may require hunters to be mobile. Hoodia gordonii helps the *Sans* sustain their energy while hunting and minimize hunger so they do not become distracted or too weak to hunt. Like the willow bark, the agents found in hoodia gordonii have been recently chemically reproduced by U.S. pharmaceutical companies and are now being sold in the United States as "P57," a diet supplement for people who want to lose weight.

Salicylic acid and hoodia gordonii are just two examples, past and recent, of contributions to Western medicine from traditional medical practices. In the following sections, we explore Chinese traditional medicine (CTM), *curanderismo* (the Mexican folk-healing practice introduced in the opening story), and Native American healing practices: three of the most widely recognized examples of traditional medicines in other cultures. We review them briefly to explore their similarities to and differences with Western medicine practices. Keep in mind, however, that the traditional practices included are a small sample of the total number of such practices, even today.

Chinese Traditional Medicine (CTM)

Chinese traditional medicine (CTM), sometimes referred to as ***traditional Chinese medicine (TCM),*** is similar to other folk medicines because it is rooted in the philosophy and the belief structure of its culture. As explained in Box 6.6, CTM consists of three main structures that, together with Chinese philosophy and nature, define an individual's well-being: yin and yang, the five elements, and Qi (pronounced ch'i).

According to Chinese philosophers, the yin–yang doctrine explains that all things function in relation to two forces, elements, or principles (Quah, 2003). These forces are in a constant state of dynamic balance, continually interacting to maintain harmony. (Harmony is a core concept in Chinese life; Quah, 2003). Thus yin and yang are complementary forces; each is needed to complete the other and to achieve and maintain harmony.

The second major structure in CTM is the ***five elements:*** metal, wood, water, fire, and earth. Each of the five elements is paired with a body organ and a season of the year, demonstrating the close connection between humans and nature. According to this philosophy, a person's health is dependent, in part, on his or her interactions with the physical environment.

The last structure, Qi, is a concept taken from Taoist philosophers. Qi is best understood as a substantial energy force that flows within the body parallel to or as part of the circulation of the blood (Quah, 2003).

TREATING ILLNESSES USING CTM To individuals unfamiliar with Chinese medicine, the philosophy of three forces that work together to influence health may be clear in concept but not in practice. Consider this: Medical providers trained in CTM are taught to probe both the physiological as well as the psychological determinants of health. Thus, instead of searching only for a proximal physical cause of an illness, health providers will explore the relationship among the affected body parts, related areas, emotional states, and physical and social environmental factors to discover the source of the disharmony.

Examining relationships among body, emotions, and nature takes time. A complete exploration of the illness and its related causes may require multiple visits as the CTM provider delves into the patient's emotional health, relationships with others in his or her family, diet, and other aspects of his or her life that may not appear to be the source of the problem but may be related to the disturbance. In this way, the CTM healing process is similar to Angelita's experience with the *curandero* in the opening story.

A principal complaint of individuals who choose the CTM approach for health care is that the process takes longer than when using Western medical methods (Lam, 2001). Still, many prefer CTM for specific ills. In a series of focus groups conducted among 29 Chinese residents of Hong Kong, Lam (2001) revealed that many believed that Western medicine is useful if seeking a quick recovery; however, they preferred CTM care when a quick Western medical treatment proved ineffective in curing the disease.

BOX 6.6 Traditional Medicines: An Overview

Chinese Traditional Medicine (CTM)

Yin and yang, the five elements, and Qi are the three principal structures of CTM. ***Yin*** is associated with passive, life-sustaining, conserving energies or latent energies that need to be actualized (Kapke, 2004; Quah, 2003). Yin energies are often associated with darkness and cold (passive, conserving energies) as well as water and females (sustaining forces). With respect to the body, yin is associated with specific organs: the heart, liver, pancreas, kidneys, and lungs. Thus, the yin organs are vital to sustaining life.

In comparison, ***yang*** energy forces are described as strong forces that cause change. They are dynamic forces that initiate action. The yang forces are usually characterized as male, consistent with the notion of males as active, assertive, or aggressive (Kapke, 2004). Thus they are associated with light, fire, heat: all active and potentially destructive forces. In the body, yang is associated with the gall bladder, small intestines, large intestines, and the bladder; organs that transmit, transform, and eliminate nonessential items from the body (Kapke, 2004). According to CTM, our health is optimal when yin and yang forces are in perfect balance. When one or the other is out of balance, however, diseases or other ailments may be present. For example, when yin is out of balance for females, a number of symptoms could appear, including irregular menstrual cycles, irritability, early menopause, or other related problems (D'Alberto, 2006).

The five elements—metal, wood, water, fire, and earth—demonstrate the relationship between human beings and nature. Specifically, these structures emphasize the role of harmony between humans and nature and their effect on well-being. Each element has both yin and yang components. For example, water evidences yin properties when it is cool and nourishing. But water also demonstrates yang energy force when it is destructive. Consider this: In a flood, objects in the path of the rushing water can be dislodged, moved, or destroyed by the pressure exerted (Kapke, 2004). Our interactions with the elements, according to CTM, will affect the balance of yin and yang in our bodies. For example, absorbing too much of the sun's rays will burn yin, the cold energy force, resulting in an imbalance and discomfort.

Finally, ***Qi*** is an energy source that flows throughout the body, similar to the body's circulatory system. The movement of Qi within the body is influenced by seasons and foods that help to facilitate or to impede its flow.

Curanderismo

Curanderos, or the traditional healers for this form of medicine, are believed to have special healing powers. It is a gift (*el don*), not something for which an individual receives formal training, as in Western medicine. Yet, most *curanderos* undergo a period of apprenticeship to learn to use their healing gifts.

Core to *curanderismo* is spirituality and maintaining harmony and balance with nature (Tafur, Crowe, & Torres, 2009). The central role of spirituality is evident in some of the more common illnesses addressed by the healers. These include *espanto*, an extreme fright believed to be caused by a supernatural force, and *susto*, a fright due to a traumatic experience (Lopez, 2005). Both illnesses are described as "soul loss" in *curanderismo* and require spiritual cures. Researchers note that *espanto* and *susto* often lead to emotional and psychological health problems, including depression, apathy, anorexia, and insomnia (Chesney et al., 2005). The spiritual causes attributed to what modern medicine considers mental health issues illustrates one contrast between traditional and Western views of health.

One similarity between *curanderismo* and Western medicine, however, is the presence of specialized practices within *curanderismo*. Like Western health practitioners, *curanderos* may be specialists. For example, herbalists (*yerberos*) focus on the treatment of physical health problems using natural herbs and homeopathic medicines. Thus stomachaches may be treated with orange leaf tea (*citrus aurantium*), earaches with garlic (*allium sativum*), or sunburns with aloe vera. Illnesses of a spiritual or supernatural origin, however, such as *susto* or *mal de ojo*, the evil eye, would be treated by an *espiritista* who would perform a *limpia* or spiritual cleansing.

Native American Healing Practices

Native American healing traditions were crucial to the survival of the first wave of colonizers to what is now the United States. In spite of this well-known history, it has taken several decades for researchers to document the Native American practices and knowledge of botany to heal both body and mind (Portman & Garrett, 2006).

Currently, there are over 500 Native American tribal nations, and so it is not possible to summarize each nation's healing practices. However, there are several core principles that apply to many Native American beliefs and practices. First, there are four constructs that are central to the healing traditions: spirituality, community, environment, and self. The core concepts of spirituality, environment, and life force are similar thematically to *curanderismo* and CTM.

Unique to the Native American practices, however, is a belief in a "circle of life" and in the concept of medicine. The circle of life symbolizes power, peace, and unity (Portman & Garrett, 2006). Each individual holds responsibility for helping to contribute to the circle by living harmoniously with all living elements that are also part of the circle.

With respect to medicines, Native American traditions contend that each person, place, and thing holds medicine within itself. To be certain, Native Americans believe in the healing powers of plants and herbs (or external agents) for holistic health needs. But consider this: Native American health beliefs hold that an event that occurred 10 years ago that made someone laugh, and that still makes that person chuckle today when recalling the incident, is a form of medicine (Portman & Garrett, 2006). The memory the person holds returns him or her to a state of well-being, if only for a moment. It provides medicine that improves one's state of well-being, if only for a limited period.

Individuals with access to both forms of medicines believe that there are additional strengths and weaknesses associated with both practices. Western medicine, in addition to being quicker, helps to rapidly control symptoms. When confronting contagious illnesses, Western medicine may be preferred for its ability to not only control the symptoms but also contain the spread of the disease. The disadvantages of Western medicine, according to the Chinese focus group participants in Lam's study, are its inability to completely cure the illness and the strong and unpleasant-tasting side effects of some of the medication.

Among users of both CTM and Western medicine, the advantages of CTM include a more effective cure for illnesses, fewer side effects, and a more effective treatment for chronic illnesses. Many prefer it as a treatment for the whole person (Hon et al., 2005; Wong et al., 2006). Finally, the fact that many users of CTM indicate that family and friends recommend the traditional method suggest that family tradition, culture, and sociological factors also influence the choice of medical approaches.

In essence, some users of CTM believe that Western medicine is the preferred approach when seeking a quick fix for a medical ailment but favor traditional medicines to treat longer-term, chronic illnesses. Consistent with Chinese philosophy, if illness represents more than just a physical disharmony, then the cure must address all elements, including the energy flow and the individual's interaction with the elements.

Curanderismo

The term *curanderismo* comes from the Spanish word *curar,* meaning to heal (Tafur, Crowe, & Torres, 2009). Like Chinese traditional medicine, *curanderismo* originated from cultural beliefs. In this case, the most immediate culture of origin is Mexican. However, anthropologists suggest that *curanderismo* has been influenced by the health beliefs and practices of the Greeks, the Moors (Arabs of northern Africa), the Aztec and Mayan empires (Krassner, 1986), and sub-Saharan African medical practices (Luna, 2003; Morales, 1998), as well as a number of European and Native American cultures (Trotter, 2001). Today, *curanderismo* is an umbrella term that refers to many types of treatments and rituals that, melded together over several centuries, represent a form of traditional healing commonly practiced in Mexico (Lopez, 2005). It is, therefore, an evolving form of medicine, continually expanding and incorporating techniques from other "folk medicines" including ***parapsychology***—here meaning psychic experiences including telepathy, clairvoyance, and psychic healing.

Central to the practice of *curanderismo* is the belief that to maintain a healthy body an individual must achieve a balance among biological needs, social-interpersonal expectations, physical and spiritual harmony, and individual and cultural-familial attachments (Vargas & Koss-Chioino, 1992). It is no surprise, therefore, that the *curandero* in the opening story looked to familial attachments and spiritual unrest as possible causes for Angelita's emotional health problems. In sum, good health, as defined by this practice, is more than freedom from illness.

Note also that, in the opening story, the *curandero* used herbs and teas as part of the healing process. Like Western health providers, many healers also have specialties (Torres & Sawyer, 2005). For example,

TABLE 6.2 Specialties in *Curanderismo*

Specialty	*Function*
Yerberos (herbalists)	Botanical remedies Homeopathic medicines Religious amulets
Partenas (midwives)	Childbirth
Sobadores (masseuses)	Massages General physical imbalances Sprains Bone setting
Espiritistas (spiritualists)	Faith healers Interpersonal relationships Spiritual health Séance

Source: Lopez (2005).

yerberos (or *yerberas,* for women) are herbalists who specialize in the use of herbs, homeopathic medicines, and religious amulets, here meaning objects or jewelry intended as protection against evil (Lopez, 2005). Given that the *curandero* in the opening story used herbs as medicinal agents, he may specialize in botanical cures.

It is important to note, however, that unlike CTM, spirituality plays a central role in the concept of health and healing in *curanderismo*. This is seen most clearly in the common types of illnesses addressed through this medicine. For example, there are a number of illnesses that are believed to be supernatural or spiritual in origin (Trotter, 2001). One such illness is *espanto,* often described as a "magical fright" because the cause of the frightened response is linked to supernatural factors. It is also linked with a loss of one's soul and as such is an ailment that is treated with spiritual cures (see Table 6.3).

In sum, *curanderismo* is a form of traditional medicine that evolved from different cultures and is still evolving today. Spirituality and spiritual forces are central to its healing practices, as is a reliance on botany to address physiological and psychological issues (see Figure 6.5).

Native American Health Practices

We must state first that there are over 500 different Native American tribal nations. Consequently, we do not imply in our heading that there is a uniform practice with respect to healing and traditional medicines for all Native Americans. As indicated at the beginning of the section on traditional medicines, here we explore the common themes among the traditional practices of the tribal nations and compare them to *curanderismo* and CTM, described previously.

Native American healing traditions have been described as a practice that involves traditional medicine practitioners—such as medicine men or women, or shamans—that is intended to restore a person to a

TABLE 6.3 Commonly Diagnosed Illnesses in *Curanderismo*

Illness	*Meaning*	*Description*	*Illnesses*
Mal aires/Mal viento	Bad air/bad winds	Illness caused by supernatural forces, exposure to sudden change in environmental temperature: cold to hot or vice-versa	Headaches, coldness, diarrhea, vomiting, paleness, fatigue
Mal de ojo	Evil eye	Supernatural or mental illness	Headaches, fever, rashes, death
Espanto/Susto	Magical fright	Illness caused by frightening experiences	Loss of soul, loss of appetite, vomiting, crying, insomnia depression, introversion
Mal projimo, duende, & brujeria	Illness caused by negative thoughts/feelings, negative encounters or witchcraft	Negative thoughts feelings of person(s) about another; negative encounters; manipulation of negative energies causing harm	Negative influences cause mental and physical harm

Sources: Cavender, A.P. & Albin, M. (2009); Lopez, R. A. (2005).

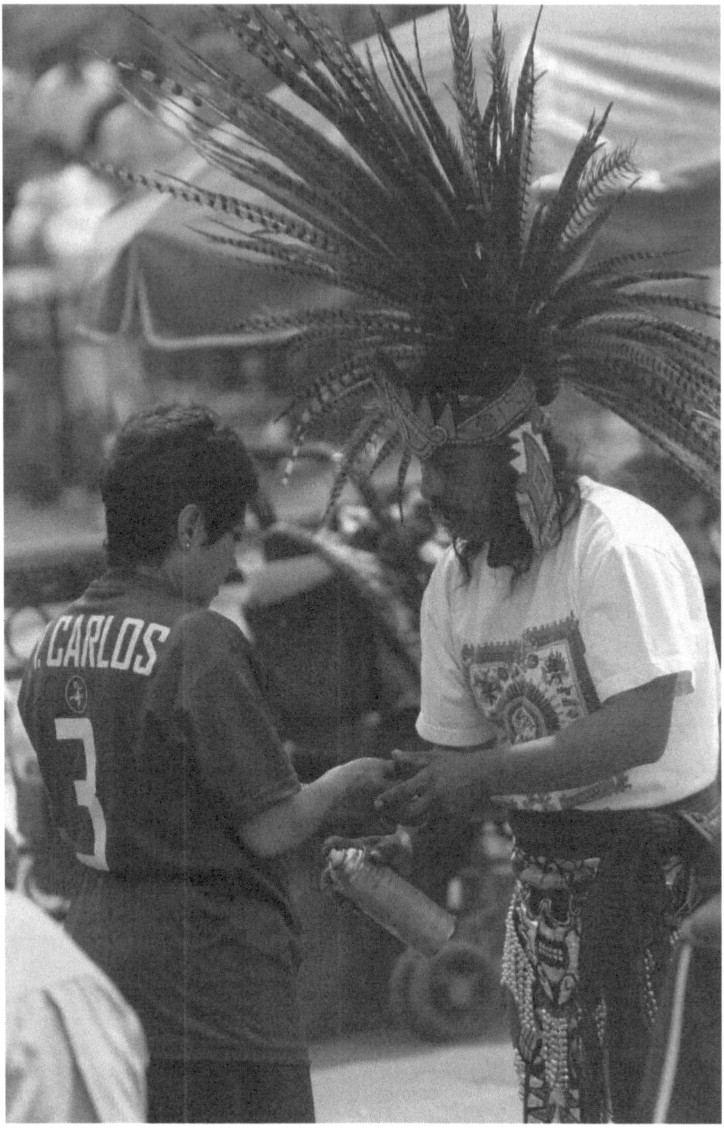

FIGURE 6.5 ***Curandero.*** Curandero with patient.

Source: Alamy B1K6YJ

healthy state (Chee, 1991). The healing process described, however, is a slow process, similar to the slow cures identified in CTM and *curanderismo*.

Principles that are common to all Native American practices are the belief in a higher power called, among other names, the Creator, the Great Spirit, or Great One; a belief in the interconnectedness of the mind, the body, and the spirit; and the belief that well-being characterizes a state of harmony among the mind, body, spirit, and natural environment (Garrett, 1998; Portman & Garrett, 2006). Native American health beliefs emphasize spirituality and the unity of mind, body, and spirit. In this way it is similar to the views expressed in *curanderismo* and more similar to the ecological model than CTM.

Not surprisingly, then, four constructs are also central to all Native American healing practices: spirituality (including the creator, Mother Earth), community (for example, family or tribe), the environment (such as nature, the land) and self (including inner passions, values, and thoughts). It is the balance among the individual, the ecological, and the spiritual that defines, for many Native Americans, "good medicine" (Portman & Garrett, 2006).

Similar to adherents of other traditional health practices, Native Americans believe that a number of forces can cause ill health. Social discord, misuse of traditional practices, and spiritual unrest are but a few of the elements that can disrupt a balance and consequently affect an individual's overall well-being.

There are, however, interesting differences in the healing practices used in this form of traditional medicine. First is the concept of medicine. Although medicinal agents can and do include herbs, teas, or pastes (poultices)—recall the example of the Disney version of Pocahontas earlier in the chapter—Native Americans believe that medicine also exists within each individual. For example, an experience that caused someone to smile and that continues to evoke the same response years later is considered medicine (Portman & Garrett, 2006). Medicine can also be the peacefulness of a moment. In essence, experiences, places, and even individuals themselves have the ability to help restore the balance between a person, the mind, the spirit, and nature.

Cohen (2003) notes interesting differences between Native American and Western medical beliefs. For example, Cohen notes that whereas Western medicine focuses on pathology and curing diseases, Native American practices, like other traditional systems, focus on healing the person and the community. Another distinction Cohen points out is the different approaches to treatment. Western medicine takes what Cohen calls an "adversarial" approach, seeking to destroy the disease. In contrast, the Native American health approach is consistent with "teological" medicine and seeks learning lessons from the disease: that is, what the person can learn or the message in the illness.

In summary, traditional medicines have existed for centuries. They continue to supply Western medicine with knowledge about the medicinal benefits of herbs and plants, the foundation for many of the prescribed or over-the-counter medicines used today. Traditional medicines retained their holistic and ecological approaches to health, focusing on the well-being of the individual, which includes physical, emotional, social, and spiritual health and harmony with one's environment. They are more consistent with an ecological model of health.

Over time, however, Western medicine's scientific-based approach to health has been refined. It retains the important contributions made by science, but now it is broadening its base to incorporate elements of traditional medical practices into its concept of health and into its treatment approaches.

Having examined "old" and "new" approaches to health, it may seem that there is nothing more to add. However, the research on stress and coping has established clear links between emotional and physical health and also demonstrates the role of social and psychological environmental factors on overall well-being. We continue the exploration of emotional health in Chapter 7, Stress and Coping.

Personal Postscript

Do you sometimes wonder about the best way to treat your chest cold, or whether you really need an antibiotic for your repeated sinus problems? If so, you might be surprised to find that people who "grew up" in a Western medicine culture are increasingly exploring alternative and complementary treatments for many recurrent illnesses.

How do you decide which method is likely to be more successful? There is no one fail-proof system for determining the most effective method. But there are a few questions you can ask to help you decide. Consider the following:

1. Is your medical care provider open to exploring alternative therapies? If not, you may want to consider seeking a second opinion from someone who is knowledgeable about alternative medicines. It would increase your options when deciding how best to treat a medical problem.
2. Is your medical problem recurrent or chronic? Have you tried a number of recommended Western treatments without much success? Perhaps now would be a time to read up on alternative therapies. You may not decide to use them, but you will educate yourself about a range of alternatives that you may consider at a later point.
3. Finally—and this may sound incredible—but is there someone in your family who has an excellent reputation for treating some acute (sudden) or chronic illnesses who had no formal medical training? Often we overlook the wisdom and collected knowledge of relatives who have acquired a wealth of information about alternative treatments. Consider obtaining your "second opinion" from that family member.

Questions to Consider

1. Increasingly, alternative and traditional forms of medicine are being used in lieu of or in conjunction with Western medical practices. What implications does this have for the work of health psychologists?
2. One reason given for excluding spirituality as a variable in health outcomes is the difficulty in measuring that factor. How would you measure spirituality?
3. The role of environment and social policy on health outcomes was explained in a study by Sir Chadwick in 1842. What examples exist today of the impact of environment and social policy on health?

Important Terms

***afferent nerve fibers* 18**
***apartheid* 36**
***aspirin* 38**
***autonomic nervous system (ANS)* 21**
***axon* 18**

References

Africa First. (2008). *Report of the Second Global Summit on HIV/AIDS, Traditional Medicine & Indigenous Knowledge*, March 10–14, 2008. Retrieved from: www.slideshare.net/andrewwilliamsjr/2008-report-re-2nd-global-summit-hivaids.

Armstrong, D. (2002). Theoretical tensions in biopsychosocial medicine. In Marks, D. (ed.) *The Health Psychology Reader*. London: Sage Publications.

Aspinwall, L. G., & Staudinger, U. M. (2003). A psychology of human strengths: Some critical issues of an emerging field. In L. G. Aspinwall & U. M. Staudinger (eds.), *A psychology of human strengths: Fundamental questions & future directions for a positive psychology* (9–22). Washington, DC: American Psychological Association.

Bjorck, J. P., Hopp, D. P., & Jones, L. W. (1999). Prostate cancer and emotional functioning: Effects on mental adjustment, optimism and appraisal. *Journal of Psychosocial Oncology*, 17(1), 71–85.

Broome, B., & Broome, R. (2007). Native Americans: Traditional healing. *Urologic Nursing*, 27(2), 161–173.

Bucko, R. A., & Cloud, S. I. (2008). Lakota health and healing. *Southern Medical Journal*, 101(6), 596–598.

Cantor, D. (2000). The diseased body. In R. Cooter & J. E. Pickstone (eds.), *Medicine in the 20th Century*. London: Harwood Press.

Carroll, D., Smith, G. D., & Bennett, P. (2002). Some observations on health and socio-economic status. In D. F. Marks (ed.), *The health psychology reader*. London: Sage Publications.

Carstensen, L. I., & Charles, S. T. (2003). Human aging: Why is even good news taken as bad? In L. G. Aspinwall & U. M. Staudinger (eds.), *A psychology of human strengths* (75–86). Washington, DC: American Psychological Association.

Cavender, A. P. & Albin, M. (2009). The use of magical plants by curanderos in the Ecuador highlands. *Journal of Ethnobiology & Ethnomedicine*, 5, 3.

Centers for Disease Control (CDC). (2008). Arthritis Types—Overview: Childhood arthritis. Retrieved from: www.cdc.gov/arthritis/arthritis/childhood.htm.

CERD Working Group on Health & Environmental Health. (2008). *Unequal health outcomes in the United States: Racial & ethnic disparities in health care treatment & access, the role of social & environmental determinants of health & the responsibilities of the state.* A Report to the U. N. Committee on the Elimination of Racial Discrimination. Accessed on September 22, 2009, from: www.prrac.org/pdf/CERDhealthEnvironmentReport.pdf.

Chadwick, Sir E. (1842). *Report from the Poor Law Commission on an Inquiry into the Sanitation Conditions of the Labouring Population of Great Britain.* United Kingdom: Craig Thornber Publisher.

Checkland, K., Harrison, S., McDonald, R., Grant, S., Campbell, S., & Guthrie, B. (2008). Biomedical, holism & general medical practice: responses to the 2004 general practitioner contract. *Sociology of Health & Wellness*, 30(5), ejournal prepublication.

Chee, V. A. (1991). Medicine men. *Journal of the American Medical Association*, 265, 17, 2276.

Chesney, M. A., Darber, L. A., Hoerster, K., Taylor, J. M., Chambers, D. B., & Anderson, D. E. (2005). Positive emotions: Explaining the other hemisphere in behavioral medicine. *International Journal of Behavioral Medicine*, 12, 2, 50–58.

Clay, R. (1977). Prevention is theme of the '98 presidential year. *The American Psychological Association Monitor.* December, 35. Washington, DC: The American Psychological Association.

Coburn, D. (2004). Beyond the income inequality hypothesis: Class, neo-liberalism, and health inequalities. *Social Science & Medicine*, 58, 41–56.

Cohen, S. (2004). Connecting social relationships and health. *Monitor on Psychology*, 35, 14–15.

Cohen, S. (2005). Keynote presentation at the Eighth International Congress of Behavioral Medicine: The Pittsburgh common cold studies: Psychosocial predictors of susceptibility to respiratory infectious illness. *International Journal of Behavioral Medicine*, 12, 3, 123–131.

Cohen, S., Doyle, W. J., Skoner, D. P., Fireman, P., Gwaltney, J. M., & Newsom, J. T. (1995). State and trait negative affect as predictors of objective and subjective symptoms of respiratory viral infections. *Journal of Personality and Social Psychology*, 68, 159–169.

Cohen, S., Kaplan, G. A., & Salonen, J. T. (1999). The role of psychological characteristics in the relations between socioeconomic status and perceived health. *Journal of Applied Social Psychology*, 29, 445–268.

Cohen, S., Tyrrell, D. A. J., & Smith, A. P. (1991). Psychological stress and susceptibility to the common cold. *New England Journal of Medicine*, 325, 606–612.

Cohen, S., Tyrrell, D. A. J., & Smith, A. P. (1993). Life events, perceived stress, negative affect and susceptibility to the common cold. *Journal of Personality and Social Psychology*, 64, 131–140.

D'Alberto, A. (2006). The withering of yin: A mid-life crisis? *Positive Health*, September, 18.

Diaz, D. P. (1993). Foundations for spirituality: establishing the variables of spirituality within the disciplines. *Journal of Health Education*, 24(6), 24–326.

Diener, E. (2000). Subjective well-being: The science of happiness and a proposal for a national index. *American Psychologist*, 55, 34–43.

Diener, E., & Suh, E. M. (2000). *Culture & subjective wellbeing*. Cambridge, MA: MIT Press.

Dinh, N. M. H., & Groleau, D. (2008). Traumatic amputation: A case of Laotian indignation and injustice. *Culture, Medicine & Psychiatry*, June 17, e-publication ahead of print.

Dusek, J. A., & Benson, H. (2009). Mind – body medium: A model of the comparative clinical impact of the acute stress & relaxation response. *Minnesota Medicine*, 92, 5, 47–50.

Engel, G. L. (2002). The need for a new medical model: A challenge for biomedicine. In D. L Marks (ed.), *The health psychology reader*. London: Sage Publications.

Folkman, S., & Greer, S. (2002). Promoting psychological well-being in the face of serious illness: When theory, research and practice inform each other. *Psychooncology*, 9, 11–19.

Gable, S. L., & Haidt, J. (2005). What (& why) is positive psychology? *Review of General Psychology*, 9, 2, 103–110.

Gallo, L. C., & Matthews, K. A. (2003). Understanding the association between socioeconomic status and physical health. Do negative emotions play a role? *Psychological Bulletin*, 129, 10–51.

Garrett, M. T. (1998). *Walking on the wind: Cherokee teachings for harmony and balance*. Santa Fe, NM: Bear & Co. Garver, C. S., Weintraub, J. K., & Scheier, M. E. (1989). Assessing coping strategies: A theoretically based approach. *Journal of Personality and Social Psychology*, 56, 267–283.

Gee, G. C., & Payne-Sturges, D. C. (2004). Environmental health disparities: A framework integrating psychosocial and environmental concepts. *Environmental Health Perspectives*, 112(17), 1645–1653.

Glassman, A. H., & Shapiro, P. A. (1998). Depression and the course of coronary artery disease. *American Journal of Psychiatry*, 155, 4–11.

Gobodo-Madikizela, P. (2002). *A human being died that night: A South African story of forgiveness*. New York: Houghton Mifflin.

Gobodo-Madikizela, P. (2003). Remorse, forgiveness & rehumanization: Stories from South Africa. *Journal of Humanistic Psychology*, 42, 1, 7–32.

Hamlin, C., & Sheard, S. (1998). Revolutions in public health: 1848–1998. *British Medical Journal*, 317, 587–591.

Held, B. S. (2002). The tyranny of positive attitudes in America: Observation and speculation. *Journal of Clinical Psychology*, 58, 9, 965–992.

Held, B. S. (2005). The "virtues" of positive psychology. *Journal of Theoretical & Philosophical Psychology*, 25, 1, 1–34.

Hon, K. L. E., Leung, T. F., Tse, H. M., Lam, L. N., Tam., K. C., & Chu, K. M. (2005). A survey of attitudes to traditional Chinese medicine among Chinese medical students. *American Journal of Chinese Medicine*, 33(2), 269–279.

Hout, M., Brooks, C., & Manzay, J. (1993). The persistence of classes in post-industrial societies. *International Sociology*, 8, 259–277.

International on Line (IOL). (2004). SA approves law to recognize sangomas. Retrieved on June 30, 2008, from: www.int.iol.co.za.

Ironson, G., & Hayward, H. (2008). Do positive psychosocial factors predict disease progression in HIV-1? A review of the evidence. *Psychosomatic Medicine*, 70(5), 546–554.

Ironson, G., Stuetzle, R., & Fletcher, M. A. (2006). An increase in religiousness/spirituality occurs after HIV diagnosis & predicts slower disease progression over four years in people with HIV. *Journal of General Internal Medicine*, 21 (Suppl. 5), S62–S68.

Jacobs, G. D. (2001). The physiology of mind – body interactions: The stress response and the relaxation response. *Journal of Alternative & Complementary Medicine*, 7, S83–92.

Jessor, R., Donovan, J. E., & Costa, F. M. (1991). *Beyond adolescence: Problem behavior and young adult development.* Cambridge, UK: Cambridge University Press.

Kapke, B. (2004). Yin & yang: Energy medicine. *Massage & Bodywork.*

Kawano, Y. (2008). Association of job-related stress factors with psychological and somatic symptoms among Japanese hospital nurses: Effects of departmental environment in acute care hospitals. *Journal of Occupational Health*, 50(1), 79–85.

Kidder, T. (2003). *Mountains beyond mountains.* New York: Random House.

Kiecolt-Glaser, J. K., & Glaser, R. (1988). Psychological influences on immunity: Implications for AIDS. *American Psychologist*, 43, 892–898.

Krassner, M. (1986). Effective features of therapy from the healer's perspective: A study of *curanderismo. Smith College Studies in Social Work*, 56, 157–183.

Lam, T. P. (2001). Strengths and weaknesses of traditional Chinese medicine and Western medicine in the eyes of some Hong Kong Chinese. *Journal of Epidemiological and Community Health*, 55, 762–762.

Lazarus, R. S. & Folkman, S. (1987). Transactional theory & research in emotions & coping. *European Journal of Personality*, 1, 141–169.

Lechner, S. C., Carver, C. S., Antoni, M. H., Weaver, K. E., & Phillips, K. M. (2006). Curvilinear associations between benefit finding & psychosocial adjustment to breast cancer. *Journal of Consulting & Clinical Psychology*, 74, 5, 828–840.

Liberatos, P., Link, B. G., & Kelsey, J. L. (1988). The measurement of social class in epidemiology. *Epidemiologic Review*, 10(1), 87–121.

Lopez, R. A. (2005). Use of alternative folk medicine by Mexican American women. *Journal of Immigrant Health*, 7, 1, 23–31.

Luna, E. (2003). *Nurse-curanderas: Las que curan* at the heart of Hispanic culture. *Journal of Holistic Nursing*, 21(4), 326–342.

Mayne, T. J. (1999) Negative effect and health: The importance of being earnest. *Cognition and Emotion*, 13, 5, 601–635.

Mizrachi, N. (2001). From causation to correlation: The story of psychosomatic medicine, 1939–1979. *Culture, Medicine & Psychiatry*, 25, 317–343.

MMWR. (2004). Alcohol-attributable deaths & years of potential life lost—United States, 2001. *MMWR*, 43, 37, 866–870. Retreived on December 29, 2008 from: www.cdc.gov/mmwr/preview/mmwrhtml/mm5337a2.htm?mobile=nocontent

Morales, A. L. (1998). *Remedios: Stories of earth and iron from the history of Puertorriquenas.* Boston: Beacon Press.

Moscowitz, J. T., Epel, E. S., & Acree, M. (2008). Positive affect uniquely predicts lower risk of mortality in people with diabetes. *Health Psychology*, 27 (1Suppl.), S73–82.

Mullen, K. D., McDermott, R. S., Gold, R. J., & Belcastro, P. A. (1996). *Connections for Health*, 4th ed. Madison, WI: Brown & Benchmark.

Myers, D. G. (2000). The funds, friends, and faith of happy people. *American Psychologists*, 55(1), 56–67.

Myslakidou, K., Tsilika, E., Parpa, E., Hatzipli, I., Smyrnioti, M., Galanos, A., et al. (2008). Demographic and clinical predictions of spirituality in advanced cancer patients: A randomized control study. *Journal of Clinical Nursing*, 17(13), 1779–1785.

Nikelly, A. G. (2005). Positive health outcomes of social interests. *Journal of Individual Psychology*, 61(4), 329–342.

Norem, J. K. (2001). Defensive pessimism, optimism & pessimism. In E. D. Chang (ed.), *Optimism & pessimism: Theory research & practice* (77–100). Washington, DC: American Psychological Association Press.

Northridge, M. E., & Sclar, E. (2003). A joint urban planning and public health framework: Contributions to health impact assessment. *American Journal of Public Health*, 93(1), 118–121.

Park, N., Peterson, C., & Seligman, M. E. P. (2004). Strengths of character & well-being. *Journal of Social and Clinical Psychology*, 23(5), 603–619.

Park, S. Y., Murphy, S. P., Sharmay, S., & Kolonel, L. N. (2005). Dietary intakes and health-related behaviors of Korean American women born in the USA & Korea: The multiethnic cohort study. *Public Health Nutrition*, 8(7), 904–911.

Pasteur, L., Chamberland, & Roux. (2002). Summary report of the experiments conducted at Pouille-le-Fort, near Melun, on the anthrax vaccination. T. Dasgupta (trans.). *Yale Journal of Biology and Medicine*, 75, 1, 59–62.

Perez-Alvarez, M> (2016). The science of happiness: As felicious as it is fallacious. *Journal of Theoretical and Philosophical Psychology*, 36, 1, 1–19.

Perrin, K. M., & McDermott, R. J. (1997). The spiritual dimension of health: A review. *American Journal of Health Studies*, 13(2), 90–99.

Peterson, C., & Seligman, M. E. P. (2004). *Character strengths & virtues: A handbook & classification*. New York: Oxford University Press.

Philpott, D. (2009). An ethic of political reconciliation. *Ethics and International Affairs*, 23, 4, 398–407.

Portman, T. A. A., & Garrett, M. T. (2006). Native American healing traditions. *International Journal of Disability, Development & Education*, 53, 4, 453–469.

Quah, S. R. (2003). Traditional healing systems and the ethos of science. *Social Science & Medicine*, 57, 1997–2012.

Rabin, B. S., Cohen, S., Ganguli, R., Lyle, D. T., & Cunnick, J. E. (1989). Bidirectional interaction between the central nervous system and immune system. *CRC Critical Reviews in Immunology*, 9(4), 279–312.

Ray, O. (2004). How the mind hurts and heals the body. *American Psychologists*, 59, 29–40.

Ryan, R. M., & Deci, E. L. (2000). Self-determination theory and the facilitation of intrinsic motivation, social development, and well-being. *American Psychologists*, 55(1), 68–78.

Salovey, P., Rothman, A. J., Detweiler, J. B., & Steward, W. T. (2000). Emotional states and physical health. *American Psychologist*, 55(1), 110–121.

Saris, W. H., Blair, S. N., vanBaak, M. A., Eaton, S. B., Davis, P. S., & DiPeitro L. (2003). How much physical activity is enough to prevent unhealthy weight gain? Outcome of the IASO 1st stock conference & consensus statement. *Obesity Review: An Official Journal of the International Association of the Study of Obesity*, 4(2), 101–114.

Schnoll, R. A., Knowles, J. C., & Harlow, L. (2002). Correlates of adjustment among cancer survivors. *Journal of Psychosocial Oncology*, 20(1), 37–59.

Schultz, A., & Northridge, M. E. (2004). Social determinants of health: Implications for environmental health promotion. *Health, Education & Behavior*, 31(4), 455–471.

Schultz, A. M., Williams, D. R., Israel, B. A., & Lempert, L. B. (2002). Racial and spatial relations as fundamental determinants of health in Detroit. *Milbank Quarterly*, 80(4), 677–707.

Schulz, R., Beach, S. R., Ives, D. G., Martire, L. M., Ariyo, A. A., & Kop, W. J. (2000). Association between depression and mortality in older adults: The cardiovascular health study. *Archives of Internal Medicine*, 160, 1761–1768.

Schulz, R., Martire, L. M., Beach, S. R., & Scheier, M. F. (2005). Depression and mortality in the elderly. In G. Miller & E. Chen E. (eds.) *Current Directions in Health Psychology*. Upper Saddle River, NJ: Prentice Hall.

Scott, P. (2007). Chronic diseases: Another challenge for the developing world. *International Journal of Clinical Practice*, 61(9), 1422–1423.

Seaward, B. L. (1991). Spiritual well-being: A health education model. *Journal of Health Education*, 22(3), 166–169. Segerstrom, S. C., & Miller, G. E. (2004). Psychological stress and the human immune system: A meta-analytic study of 30 years of inquiry. *Psychological Bulletin*, 130, 4, 601–630.

Seligman, M. E. P. (2002). Positive psychology, positive prevention & positive therapy. In C. R. Snyder & J. Shane J. (eds.), *Handbook of positive psychology* (3–9). New York: Oxford University Press.

Seligman, M. E. P., & Csikszentmihalyi, M. (2000). Positive psychology. *American Psychologist*, 55, 5–14.
Seligman, M. E. P., Park, N., & Peterson, C. (2004). The value in action (VIA) classification of character strength. *Ricechi di Psicologia*, 27, 1, 63–78.
Seligman, M. E. P., Steen, T. A., Park, N., & Peterson, C. (2000). Positive psychology in progress. *American Psychologist*, 60(5), 410–421.
Sheldon, K. M., & King, L. (2001). Why positive psychology is necessary. *American Psychologist*, 56, 216–217.
Simon, A. E., Chan, K. S., & Forrest, C. B. (2008). Assessment of children's health-related quality of life in the United States with a multidimensional index. *Pediatrics*, 121, 1, e118–e126.
Sundararajan, L. (2005). Happiness donut: A Confucian critique of positive psychology. *Journal of Theoretical & Philosophical Psychology*, 25, 1, 35–60.
Tafur, M. M., Crowe, T. K., & Torres, S. E. (2009). A review of *curanderismo* and healing practices among Mexicans and Mexican Americans. *Occupational Therapy International*, 16, 1, 82–88.
Tan, S. Y., & Berman, E. (2008). Robert Koch (1843–1910): Father of microbiology & Nobel laureate. *Singapore Journal of Medicine*, 49, 11, 854–855.
Taylor, S. E., Klein, L., Lewis, B., Gruenewald, T., Gurung, R., Updegraff, J. (2000). Biobehavioral responses to stress in females: tend-and-befriend, not fight-or-flight. *Psychological Review*, 107, 411–429.
Taylor, J., & Turner, R. J. (2001). A longitudinal study of the role and significance of mattering to others for depressive symptoms. *Journal of Health and Social Behavior*, 42, 310–325.
Taylor, S. E., Kemeny, M. E., Reed, G. M., Bower, J. E., & Gruenewald, T. L. (2000). Psychological resources, positive illusions, and health. *American Psychologists*, 55(1), 99–109.
Thompson, W., & Hickey, J. (2005). *Society in focus*. Boston: Allen & Bacon.
Torres, E., & Sawyer, T. (2005). *Curanderismo: A life in Mexican folk healing*. Albuquerque: University of New Mexico Press.
Toye, F. M., Barlow, J., Wright, C., & Lamb, S. E. (2006). Personal meanings in the construction of need for total knee replacement surgery. *Social Science and Medicine*, 63, 43–53.
Trotter, R. T. (2001). *Curanderismo:* A picture of Mexican-American folk healing. *Journal of Alternative and Complementary Medicine*, 7(2), 129–131.
UNICEF. (2008). UNICEF nominee Paul Farmer receives CDC foundation hero Award. Retrieved on February 23, 2009, from: www.unicef.org/infobycountry/usa_45896.html.
University of Arkansas, Division of Agriculture. (2007). *Natural resources. Uses of other tree species*. Retrieved on June 26, 2008, from: www.arnatural.org/wildfoods/uses_Trees.htm.
Vargas, L. A., & Koss-Chioino, J. D. (eds.). (1992). *Working with culture: Psycho-therapeutic interventions with ethnic minority children and adolescents*. San Francisco: Jossey-Bass.
Wachholtz, A. B., & Pargament, K. I. (2008) Migraines and meditation: Does spirituality matter? *Journal of Behavioral Medicine*, 31(4), 351–366.
Wade, D. T., & Halligan, P. W. (2004). Do biomedical models of illness make for good healthcare systems? *British Medical Journal*, 329, 1398–1491.
Walda, I. C., Tabak, C., Smit, H. A., Rasanen, L., Fidanza, F., Menotti, A., et al. (2002). Diet & 20 year chronic obstructive pulmonary disease mortality in middle-aged men from three European countries. *European Journal of Clinical Nutrition*, 56(7), 638–643.
Wilkinson, R. G. (1996). *Unhealthy societies: The afflictions of inequality*. London: Routledge.
Williams, R., & Williams, V. (1993). *Anger kills*. New York: Random House.
Wong, W. C. W., Lee, A., Wong. S. Y. S., Wu, A. C., & Robinson, N. (2006). Strengths, weaknesses, and development of traditional medicine in the health system of Hong Kong: Through the eyes of future Western doctors. *Journal of Alternative and Complementary Medicine*, 12(2), 185–189.
World Health Organization (WHO). (2002). World Health Organization Report: Reducing risk, promoting healthy lives. Geneva: WHO.
World Health Organization (WHO). (2003). *Traditional medicine*. Fact sheet No. 134. Retrieved from: www.who.int/mediacentre/factsheets/fs134/en/.
Yang, E. J., Chung, H. K., Kim, W. Y., Bianchi, L., & Song, W. O. (2007). Chronic diseases & dietary changes in relation to Korean American's length of residence in the United States. *Journal of the American Dietetic Association*, 107(6), 942–950.

2

STRESS AND COPING

On being well in yourself

This chapter was first published in *The Psychology of Wellbeing* and cross-referencing relates to chapters in the original volume. Please visit www.routledge.com/9780367898083 for more information about the book

NO RETURN?

A graffito on a wall in Hong Kong during the coronavirus pandemic read, 'We can't return to normal because the normal we had was precisely the problem'.

Burnout due to overwork is a universal problem. But legislation, when it exists, more often applies to physical hazards, rather than psychological ones.[1] In 2019, a survey on work-related stress, published by the Health and Safety Executive, found there were 602,000 workers in the UK suffering from anxiety and depression. This led to 12.8 million working days lost, and the main causes cited – which are consistent over time – were workload, lack of support, and coping with change.[2] In the US, stress related to discrimination and poverty costs the US economy around $300 billion every year, in accidents, absenteeism, employee turnover, reduced productivity, and medical, legal, and insurance costs.[3]

When the World Health Organization (WHO) definition of health is 'complete physical, mental and social wellbeing', any deviation from perfection could be 'abnormal', and so needs to be fixed. But are any of us, ever, completely 'well in ourselves'?[4] Whatever the 'new normal' will look like, we can start by examining the old one. And part of that is asking, is stress always a bad thing?

In this chapter, we consider the question 'what is normal?' We explore the tension between survival and growth and consider differ models of defining and coping with stress.

WHAT IS NORMAL WELLBEING?

A matter of adjustment?

'Normal' is not so easy to define. And we don't question it, until our behaviour or that of others flouts unspoken rules. And yet, normality is another idea central to our wellbeing.

In his poem *The Unknown Citizen*, composed in 1939, W.H. Auden gives us a eulogy by a government bureaucrat to a model citizen.[5] The poem is in the form of a dystopian report gathered from the data sources of a hyper-vigilant, totalitarian state. The poem ends with the lines:

> *Was he free? Was he happy? The question is absurd:*
> *Had anything been wrong, we should certainly have heard.*

Throughout the poem, Auden touched on one of the main criteria for psychological normality. But underpinning it all, based on an unremarkable life, the man is judged a saint, based on his conformity, compliance, and predictability. And questions of freedom and happiness are meaningless. Psychiatrist Robert Lindner, in his criticisms of psychology and therapy, argue that they are tools of adjustment. But he doesn't see this as a good thing. He rails, 'Corralled in body an enervated in spirit by these delegated, elected, or self-appointed herdsmen of humanity, our society has been seized and help captive by the delusion that adjustment is the whole life, its ultimate good'.[6] For Linder, the 11th commandment is 'thou shalt adjust'. Are you normal? And how do you know? Let's consider several criteria we can use to answer those questions.

Normality – where do we draw the line?

There are several ways theories in psychology define normal. We can use statistics, societal norms, positive mental health, levels of personal distress, and maladaptiveness.

Statistical criterion

In psychology we assume that most human traits and characteristics confirm to the normal distribution. It's informally called a 'bell curve' because of its shape. In the absence of a diagram, it helps to compare it to 'Anne Elk's theory of Brontosauruses' from *Monty Python's Flying Circus*.[7] Her 'theory' states, 'All brontosauruses are thin at one end, much, much thicker in the middle, and then thin again at the far end'. And, so is the normal distribution. If we imagine a line running down the thickest part of the beast (or the peak of the bell curve), that's the average – the mean. This is the measure of central tendency for the range of scores. And in statistics we also need a measure of the spread of the scores. This is known as the standard deviation. One standard deviation either side the mean accounts for around 68%. And two standard deviations either side the mean accounts for 95%. This percentage we'd consider to be normal, given variations due to individual differences. That leaves the 2.5% at the extreme ends (the head and the tail). But the statistical criterion is neutral. It doesn't distinguish between atypical behaviour that is desirable versus undesirable – such as a creative genius versus the disturbed despot. Just because most people do it doesn't make it desirable or that they ought to do it.

Deviation from the norm

A deviation from 'the norm' implies a sense of oughtness – not behaving as one should. It's usually judged by external standards, such as society, culture, community, organization, or family. It is the need to meet certain expectations, or our perception of them.

Handwashing after we've been to the toilet has an oughtness, and we'd hope it would be the norm. During the COVID-19 crisis, we have been bombarded with reminders to do it and how to do it. From a statistical perspective, we'd expect a 95% compliance rate, but in a pre-pandemic survey of European habits, only two countries, Bosnia and Herzegovina (96%) and Moldova (94%), hit the mark.[8] At the bottom of the table of compliance, some countries were around the 50% mark (mentioning no names). But post-pandemic with 'the new normal' we might see fewer differences between countries. There are different norms within countries, between countries, and throughout history. During the pandemic lockdown, anxiety, stress, and boredom were the norm. And in some societies, sexism, racism, and homophobia were the norm, and probably still are to a less blatant degree. In some, they definitely are. And as we discussed in Chapter Three, when viewed through an intersectional lens, there are norms which we accept for others that we would not accept for ourselves.

Positive mental health

Social psychologist Marie Jahoda's 1958 book *Current Concepts of Positive Mental Health* is often relegated to a paragraph in introductory psychology textbooks. And the criticisms they offer are more to do with a misreading of the original book.[9] The idea behind the book was to gather the main strands of the various theories of positive mental health. She found six major categories of concepts from an extensive literature review.[10]

There are:

1. *Attitudes of the individual towards the self* – this included a realistic sense of selfhood in relation to goals and objectives. A sense of the real-self versus the ideal-self, and self-acceptance.
2. *Growth, development, or self-actualization* – to aspire to reach one's full potential. Interest and motivation to reach future goals.
3. *Integration of psychological functions* (incorporating 1 and 2) – a balance of conscious and unconscious forces, and to resist and cope with stress.

4 *Autonomy* – self-determination and independence. That is, overly ruled by environmental factors.
5 *Adequate perception of reality* – this means relative freedom from need-distortion, or in order words, not distorting information to how you want to see it. Also, having empathy and social sensitivity.
6 *Environmental mastery* – this includes achievement in some areas of life, adequate functioning in the world (focus on process – getting along). Examples of these include (a) the ability to love; (b) adequacy in love, work, interpersonal relations, and play; (c) efficiency in meeting situational requirements; (d) capacity for adaptation and adjustment; (e) efficiency in problem solving.

Of course, judging by these standards, none of us is normal – they are a collection of ideals. But we can see here a prototype for models of human flourishing in psychology.

In another of Jahoda's works on unemployment, she identified five factors vital to wellbeing that stem from being employed. We can apply these to the destabilizing effects of the lockdown during the COVID-19 pandemic. During this time many people experienced a loss of time structure, social contact, collective effort or purpose, social identity or status, and regular activity.[11] However, a main criticism of Jahoda's work is the Western-centrism. In her review of positive mental health, many of the concepts have meaning in individualistic societies, more so than in collectivist ones. And running throughout is the assumption that good mental health and wellbeing depend on adjustment and productivity.

As Jahoda's findings mentioned the self quite extensively, social psychologist Michael Argyle cites four major factors which influence the development of the self and how we evaluate it (our self-esteem):

1 The ways in which others (particularly significant others) react to us – whether people admire us, flatter us, seek out our company, listen attentively, agree with us, avoid us, neglect us, tell us things about ourselves that we don't want to hear.

2 How we think we compare to others – favourable versus unfavourable comparisons.
3 Our social roles – some carry prestige and others carry a stigma. Some carry power and others are powerless.
4 The extent to which we identify with other people – roles aren't just 'out there'. They also become part of our personality, so that we identity with the positions we occupy, the roles we play, and the groups we belong to.

Personal distress

A key definition of normality is a subjective feeling of personal distress. It might not be obvious to outsiders because we might keep such feelings hidden. Signs of personal distress can be both psychological and physical. We might feel miserable, depressed, or agitated. Also, it might disturb sleep patterns and appetite and manifest in aches and pains.

When I have initial consultations with potential clients, it is common for them to ask whether coaching or counselling would be the best way forward. I ask questions to find out the level of personal distress. If their issues have a strong emotional part, then I can refer them on to colleagues in counselling of psychotherapy. Coaching is more about development goals.

Maladaptiveness

Sometimes people are judged 'abnormal' if their behaviour adversely affects their own wellbeing or that of others – physically, psychologically, or both. The concept is of being a risk to one's own or others' wellbeing or safety. Through the various definitions of normality there's a tension between 'fitting in' and 'just getting by' and the need to thrive and excel.

SURVIVAL VERSUS GROWTH

If you've ever attended a training workshop, it's unlikely you have avoided 'Maslow's Hierarchy of Needs'.[12] It's usually presented as a pyramid, with 'self-actualization' at the peak – the idea that you can 'be the best possible version of you' – that's how self-help books describe it. And although it's overused, it offers a useful thread to link inequalities (from the earlier chapter) and stress.

- *Self-actualization*: realizing personal potential, self-fulfilment, seeking personal growth and peak experiences.
- *Aesthetic*: appreciation and search for beauty, balance, and form.
- *Cognitive*: knowledge and understanding, curiosity, exploration, need for meaning and predictability.
- *Esteem*: ego and status needs, and the need for recognition and to be valued.
- *Love and social belongingness*: family life, friendships, relationships, and intimacy.
- *Safety and security*: money, a job, health, and a safe environment.
- *Physiological*: food, water, sleep, and shelter – the basics to function/exist.

So as we move towards the top of the list we have growth needs, and as we move towards the bottom we have survival needs. We might call these basic needs the Four Fs (feeding, fighting, fleeing and 'copulating'). And the theory is that we need to satisfy the basic needs before we can satisfy the higher needs. Stress can occur at any level, depending on the pressures we face, the goals we have, and our resources to deal with them. We might experience frustration and conflicts, a disruption of bodily rhythms, life changes, daily hassles, or just the way we habitually deal with problems.

Psychiatrist Robert Lindner argues that our struggle to reach our full potential (or just survive) is a constant source of stress. According to him, we must conquer the 'triad of limitations' that forms our prison cell. 'One side is the medium by which we must live, the second is the equipment we have or can fashion with which to live, and the third is the fact of our mortality'.[13] It's bleak, but it resonates with the definition of wellbeing from the introduction – a state of balance between challenges and resources.[14] So, is wellbeing just the absence of stress?

WHAT IS STRESS?

How we conceive of stress determines how we respond and adapt to it, and how we cope with it. And we can advance three models of stress, each from a different angle:[15]

- *Stimulus* – stress is what happens to us.
- *Response* – stress is what happens inside us.
- *Transaction* – stress is what happens between us.

Stimulus – what causes stress?

In 1967, two psychiatrists, Thomas Holmes and Richard Rahe, created the *Social Readjustment Rating Scale* (SRRS). It consists of 43 life events, each scored to reflect the degree of adjustment it might need to get over them. These life events include the death of loved ones, divorce, personal injury, illness, losing one's job, trouble with the boss, and moving to a new house. It also covers marriage, retirement, gaining a new member of the family, and holidays. And it looks at changes in habits such as diet or sleep patterns. The scores of each event range from 11 to 100 and the total score is between 11 and 600. A score of more than 300 indicates a high risk of becoming ill.[16]

For Holmes and Rahe, stress in an independent variable that acts upon the individual. And although higher SRRS scores correlate with illness, the association is quite small. But there are several criticisms of the theory. It assumes that change is inherently stressful, and that life events demand the same level of adjustment for everyone. It also assumes a common threshold beyond which illness will result. Furthermore, it sees a person as a passive recipient of stress. Later advances in the theory include the role of the individual's interpretation of life events.[17] But, the model still ignores the effects of life experience, learning, environment, and personality. However, the SRRS is still useful as a basis for discussion in a therapeutic situation or for chats among family and friends.

Response – how we react to stress

In his best-selling book *The Stress of Life*, published in 1956, endocrinologist Hans Selye outlines his general adaptation syndrome (GAS).[18] According to his theory, stress is a defensive mechanism and follows three stages: alarm, resistance, and exhaustion.

Gas: the three stages

Alarm: This refers to the first symptoms your body experiences in response to stress. The sympathetic nervous system activates these changes to prepare to combat or avoid the stressor (fight or flight).[19]Your heart rate increases, your adrenal gland releases cortisol (a stress hormone), glucose, and you get a boost of adrenaline, which increases energy.

Resistance: In this stage, if the stress is not removed the body begins to recover from the alarm reaction and to cope with the situation. Your body stays on higher alert and resists the stressor. If you overcome the stress or it ceases to be a problem, your body continues to repair itself. And your hormone levels, heart rate, and blood pressure return to pre-alarm states. In this stage you might experience irritability, frustration, and poor concentration. The parasympathetic nervous system restores returns physiological levels to normal. Also, this system causes the 'freeze' response in the body so that you feel unable to act or move.

Exhaustion: This stage is the result of chronic stress – struggling with stress for extended periods. It drains your physical, emotional, and mental resources. It can result in fatigue, disturbed eating patterns, anxiety, burnout, and depression. Physically, chronic stress impairs the immune system, making us less able to fight off attacks from bacteria and virus. It is also associated with asthma, colitis, and ulcers and is implicated in heart attacks and cancer. In fact, chronic stress has a negative effect on all bodily systems.[20]

It is neither possible nor desirable to remove every stressor from our lives. But if we spot the early warning signs for us, we can take steps to manage stress levels and lower our risk of the more serious conditions. Exercise, breathing exercises, laughing, and meditation can help your body to recover at the resistance stage and keep stress at a healthier level.[21]

What is healthy stress?

In *The Stress Concept: Past, Present and Future*, published in 1983, Selye distinguishes between bad stress, which he calls *distress*, and the good stuff: *eustress*. What we commonly call stress is distress, when we get a 'shut-down' of higher level thinking as we focus on basic survival needs (The Four Fs). In constrast, eustress is marked by focused attention and enhanced performance. Many of us need the threat of a deadline to get us started on a task.[22] This classification follows on from the Yerkes-Dodson law.[23] For complex, unfamiliar, or difficult tasks, we need moderate levels of stress for optimal performance. Without any stress we remain unmotivated, but when overwhelmed our performance declines.

Transaction – how do we cope with stress?

The transactional model sees stress arising between people and their environment. One problem with the SRRS is most of the 43 life events are not daily events. To explain stress as a more dynamic (and everyday) process, psychologists Richard Lazarus and Susan Folkman advanced the transactional theory of stress and coping. They define psychological stress as 'a particular relationship between the person and the environment that is appraised by the person as taxing or exceeding his or her resources and endangering his or her wellbeing'.[24] The appraisal is a process of categorizing any encounter in how it is likely to affect wellbeing.

The model applies two levels of appraisal, and then a choice of coping strategy:

- *First appraisal of the event* – Is it insignificant? Is it desirable or likely to benefit me? Or am I in trouble? Is it a threat, a challenge, or a loss?

(Here we might misperceive a trivial event as a threat.) Also, there's an appraisal of whether the challenge might become a benefit.
- *Second appraisal* – Do I have the resources for how to deal with the negative event to ensure a positive outcome? Can I cope with this situation? If not, a negative stress reaction occurs. Resources can be physical, social, psychological, or material. (Here we might not accurately assess our resources or lack confidence in our ability to cope.)
- *Coping strategy* – Based on the second appraisal we use either emotion-focused or control-focused strategies.

Emotion-focused coping

Emotion-focused coping involves trying to reduce the negative emotional responses associated with stress, such as sadness, fear, or frustration. If the stress is outside your control, then it might be your only option. Some of these strategies are quick fixes and can become habits, which also lead to stress. We might use food, distraction (watching TV), exercise, journaling (writing down thoughts), prayer, mindfulness, breathing techniques, or talking to someone (friends, therapist, coach). A therapeutic intervention can include a new cognitive appraisal of the stressful event. Of course, other emotion-focused strategies include alcohol, drugs, and gambling.[25] If you experience a bully in the workplace, start to keep a diary to deal with the emotion, which might later become evidence as part of a problem-solving strategy.

Control-focused coping

Control-focused strategies attempt to go to the source of the issue, such as problem solving, time management, new learning or training, and getting support, mentoring, or coaching.[26] This might also include getting more information to re-evaluate the problem. It might also include recourse to formal complaint procedures, or legal remedies. Other strategies include reading a book or controlling the amount of bad news you attend to.[27]

Another transactional model of stress involves taking control of the small stuff on a daily basis.

EVERYDAY HASSLES AND UPLIFTS

Psychologist Allen Kanner and colleagues[28] proposed a theory of stress based on the petty hassles we meet, such as losing keys, spilling drinks, or encounters with rude people. They composed a *Hassles Scale* of 117 items. They balanced this with an *Uplifts Scale* of 135 items, such as getting on well with people, receiving compliments, or just generally feeling good that day. In a study lasting over 12 months, the researchers found that hassles predicted negative psychological symptoms of stress, and hassles were a stronger predictor than that measured by the SRRS (major life events). One finding, useful for coaching, is that major life events, such as divorce, exert stress by several daily hassles. These including managing money, eating alone, or simply having to tell people about it.[29] And this everyday approach has two main benefits. First, it helps to break down major stressful events into manageable goals for control-focused coping, which, second, helps to tackle physical symptoms as they occur.

At the end of each day we do a mental balance sheet. If hassles outweigh the uplifts, we say we've had 'a bad day'. And for the opposite, we call it a good day. And the benefit of this approach is we can keep a check on the day to neutralize hassles and create our own uplifts.

And this idea of 'control what you can as you go' is a central theme in the idea of how some people manage change better than do others.

PSYCHOLOGICAL HARDINESS

Psychologists Suzanne Kobasa and Salvatore Maddi propose a combination of attitudes that creates a buffering effect against stress. Initially they studied male business executives to find out why some developed health problems while others remained healthy. And over the years the buffer effect has been shown in a large variety of groups including the military, firefighters, and university staff and students.

The three attitudes of hardiness have a moderating effect on stress by encouraging effective mental and behavioural coping, building and using social support, and practising self-care. Rather than a personality characteristic, it is more of an explanatory style – a series of attitudes (the three Cs) that shape our view of the world:[30]

- *Commitment* – 'a predisposition to be involved with people, things, and contexts rather than be detached, isolated, or alienated'.
- *Control* – 'struggling to have an influence on outcomes going on around oneself, rather than sinking into passivity and powerlessness'.
- *Challenge* – 'wanting to learn continually from experience positive or negative rather than trying to play it safe by avoiding uncertainties and potential threats'.

Maddi stresses the importance of adopting all three attitudes and not letting one dominate. Individuals 'high in hardiness' are more likely to put stressful life events into perspective and tend to perceive them as less of a threat and more of a challenge and as opportunities for personal development. Consequently, stressful events are less likely to impact negatively on a person's health.

In my coaching practice and confidence-building workshops, I use the three Cs to encourage clients to set small meaningful goals – to reach out and show curiosity about the world, to take stock of the small things that are already in their control, and to break down a larger problem into smaller challenges.

LIFE SKILLS/LEARNING SKILLS

In my professional practice I run a workshop, *Learning Skills as Life Skills (and Vice Versa)*, which illustrates how we can bring together all aspects of psychology to improve wellbeing and enhance performance. It is a modified structure from my study skills book, *Letters to a New Student*.[31]

It offers a model to flourish in education as in life and draws on transactional theories of stress and control-focused coping. It's tempting to view formal education as learning and then everything else that happens afterwards as your 'real life'. However, it's a false dichotomy. We continue to learn throughout our lives, whether we want to or not. How we approach learning informs how we approach life and vice versa. I offer four interacting factors as a blueprint for lifelong learning: *attitudes*, *wellbeing*, *cognition*, and *management*. A change in one can have a knock-on effect in the others.

Attitudes

Attitudes are the cornerstone of how we make sense of the world. In coaching, I use the tenet 'the viewing influences the doing, and vice versa'. It's a key principle in confidence building that emphasizes the link between thoughts, feeling, and actions. How we view the world shapes what we do in the world.[32] The main strand in this factor is psychological hardiness – the three Cs.

Wellbeing

Wellbeing is a strong theme in the book, and is related to how we can reduce stress, improve mood, and boost cognition. The idea is to lay the foundations and give yourself a head start when studying. The wellbeing factor includes diet and hydration, exercise, sleep, and relaxation exercises and how they interact. When we feel stressed, these are often the first things we sacrifice. I'll outline, briefly, some of the intersections and how they support learning (and life in general).

- *Diet*. A healthy (no junk food) diet has a positive impact on gut bacteria (the microbiome), which helps us to absorb nutrients from food. As most of our serotonin ('the happy chemical') is made in the gut, a poor diet can inhibit it and lower mood and can be linked to anxiety. Although the research on hydration is mixed, some studies show that low hydration can impair cognition.[33]

- *Exercise.* We can boost cognition with just 20 minutes of aerobic activity, and this can also help improve your sleep. Exercise can also lift our mood, and short bursts of physical activity are useful in releasing stress and providing a break during long work periods.[34]
- *Sleep.* Unsatisfying sleep and disturbed routines have a negative knock-on effect for diet, and you'll be more drawn to junk food. Also, sleep loss can impair cognition and lower your mood.[35]
- *Relaxation.* Breathing exercises and meditation practice can help to reduce stress so that it stays in the 'eustress range' to improve performance.[36]

Cognition

The basis for efficient learning is to work with principles of psychology instead of working against them. This approach includes short but intense study periods and creating variety in study plans to appeal to all the senses, as well as leading your reading with questions to deepen understanding instead of using surface tactics like rote learning.[37] We look at a method of active reading in the next chapter when we consider how to make the most of a self-help book.

Management

Making the effort, actively, to manage moods, emotions, time, and resources will support the learning process. It's also about recognizing that boredom is a choice. We have the resources to tackle this negative attitude and create variety and contextual cues to improve cognition. Part of this is setting goals and using control-focused coping strategies rather than being ruled by our emotions, and part of managing learning and life is knowing when to ask for support and where to get it.[38]

MORE ON COPING WITH STRESS

Does mindfulness work?

Mindfulness is defined as 'the awareness that arises from paying attention, on purpose, in the present moment, and non-judgmentally'.[39] It is often touted as the panacea for all ills. But is it? Well, the short answer is no. The evidence-based answer is more nuanced. First, the basic principle in psychology for treating anxiety disorders is that anxiety and relaxation cannot co-exist.[40] And, relaxation techniques for part of the core psychological skills for elite performance in sports psychology.[41] So, there is a basis on which to suppose that mindfulness techniques have a beneficial effect.

A review of the research on the outcomes of mindfulness practices concludes that there is convincing evidence to show that they do help to lower stress, anxiety, and depression. And there are mixed findings on its effects to improve memory and attention. It has been effective when combined with psychotherapy, such as mindfulness-based cognitive therapy (MBCT) for recurring depression. Although, it's no more effective than other forms of psychotherapy. However, in non-clinical settings, such as schools and the workplace, results are more mixed. It depends on how mindfulness is used, and how well the studies are devised. There's also evidence of publication bias that favours positive results, which might exaggerate the effects of mindfulness.[42] So there is cause for some caution, but overall there is sound enough evidence to support the use of mindfulness as part of a holistic plan to deal with stress, as described earlier. But mindfulness on its own will not help to tackle the root of the problem, just our reactions. In many cases, that might be enough, but maybe we need to change the narrative. What if we challenged the Western appropriation of mindfulness and instead restore its own psychological roots. What if we used it in pursuit of a new normal to critique capitalism and consumerism?

Taking cures

Clinical psychologist Stephen Briers writes, 'people come into therapy . . . because they instinctively feel that the stories they have sought to live by are unravelling'.[43] Sometimes events can undermine our sense of self and challenge the narratives we hold to be true. Sometimes we entertain a number of self-stories that compete and conflict. Or we might find ourselves cast in a role we didn't chose or feel powerless to escape.[44] Left unchecked, chronic (long-term) stress can lead to anxiety and depression, and so in Briers's terms, therapy can help to 'forge a new narrative . . . one that reinterprets the past or opens up new possibilities for the future'.[45] But which 'talking cures' work best?

The equivalence paradox

When we look at the research comparing the outcomes from different types of therapy, one clear finding emerges. It's called the equivalence paradox. And it is best summed up by the verdict of the Dodo Bird in *Alice in Wonderland*: 'Everyone has one and all must have prizes'.[46] In other words, they all perform much the same. And these findings have been consistent since the 1930s. So no, cognitive-behavioural therapy (CBT) is not the answer to everything either, despite the hype.[47]

We can attribute a large part of the therapeutic effect to 'common factors', such as the relationship with the therapist (30%), and placebo, hope, and expectancy (15%). The specific techniques and models explain 15% of the treatment variance. And the largest factor, which accounts for 40%, is for the personal resources and life circumstances of the client.[48]

Finding help

The most important thing is to make sure you seek out a qualified therapist. Every country has accreditation bodies for psychotherapy, counselling, and coaching, and each has guidance on what questions to ask. However, many of the practical considerations are determined by how the sessions are funded. When funded by employers, health insurance, or a referral from your doctor, it tends to be for a fixed number of sessions. You are also unlikely to be given any choice in the type of intervention. However, research indicates that the optimal number of sessions is between four and ten. And surprisingly, the median number of therapy sessions is just one. We are not sure whether therapy didn't suit these clients, or whether one session was all it took to make a difference.[49] Finally we consider thoughts of a new normal. And this shift is not necessarily a new post-pandemic normal. That's likely to take time. It might just be something that's 'new to you'.

TOWARDS A NEW NORMAL

As the UK prepared to ease lockdown restrictions, writer Matt Haig tweeted, 'Yes lockdown poses its own mental health challenges. But can we please stop pretending our former world of long working hours, stressful commutes, hectic crowds, shopping centres, infinite choice, mass consumerism, air pollution and 24/7 everything was a mental health utopia'.[50] Haig has spoken and written about his own mental health. And his two self-help-type books seem quite appropriate for post-pandemic reflection: *Reasons to Stay Alive* and *Notes on a Nervous Planet*. Also, it's noteworthy that book sales massively increased during lockdown. And we know that reading lowers stress.[51] So, more books might be part of the new normal.

The COVID-19 pandemic has offered us an opportunity to pause, reflect, and take stock of attitudes, beliefs, behaviour, and routines. What insights do you have on your ability to adapt your thoughts, emotions, and behaviour as the situation demands? How has your understanding of yourself and others changed for relationships, communication, and social awareness? What small things can you control to make a difference? What power or influence do you have over the lives of others?[52] Of all the changes you had to make, what's worth hanging on to?

SUMMARY AND REFLECTION

In this chapter we:

- explored several criteria for normal in the context of wellbeing
- considered three ways in which to understand stress, that is, as a stimulus, as a response and as a transaction. mechanisms.
- looked at life skills as learning skills and how to cope with stress.

How has the information in this chapter affected your idea of 'normal wellbeing'? And what might a 'new normal' look like, for you?

In the next chapter we explore the self-help industry, including how to choose and use a self-book.

NOTES

1 Wheeler Johnson, M. (2013). Burnout Is Everywhere – Here's What Countries Are Doing to Fix It. *Huff Post*. See: www.huffingtonpost.co.uk/entry/worker-burnout-worldwide-governments_n_3678460?ri18n=true. Accessed 1/4/2020.
2 Work-related stress, anxiety or depression statistics in Great Britain (2019). Health and Safety Executive. See: www.hse.gov.uk/statistics/causdis/stress.pdf. Accessed 19/4/2020.
3 Mohney, G. (2018). Stress Costs U.S. $300 Billion Every Year. *Healthline*. See: www.healthline.com/health-news/stress-health-costs#1. Accessed 19/4/2020. And: Brondolo, E., Byer, K., Gianaros, P.J., Liu, C., Prather, A.A., Thomas, K. & Woods-Giscombé, C.L. (2017). Stress and Heath Disparities. Contexts, Mechanisms, and Interventions Among Racial/Ethnic Minority and Low Socioeconomic Status Populations. American Psychological Association. www.apa.org/pi/health-disparities/resources/stress-report.pdf. Accessed 25/4/2020.
4 Misselbrook, D. (2014). W Is for Wellbeing and the WHO Definition of Health. *British Journal of General Practice*, 64 (628), p. 582. See: www.ncbi.nlm.nih.gov/pmc/articles/PMC4220217/. Accessed 21/4/2020.
5 Poem: 'The Unknown Citizen' by W.H. Auden (1907–1973). Poets.org: See: https://poets.org/poem/unknown-citizen. Accessed 17/4/2020. I had hoped to reproduce the poem but did not receive a reply in time for permission to use it.
6 Lindner, R. (1952, 1971). *The Revolutionist's Handbook*. New York: Grove Press, p. 67.
7 Sketch from Episode 32. The show ran from 1969 to 1974 on BBC TV.
8 Sims, A. (2015). The European Countries That Wash Their Hands Least After Going to the Toilet. *The Independent*. See: www.independent.co.uk/news/world/europe/the-european-countries-that-wash-their-hands-least-after-going-to-the-toilet-a6757711.html. Accessed 25/4/2020. See also: Timins, H. (2020). Hands Down, Men Worse at Bathroom Hygiene That Prevents Coronavirus. *Reuters*. www.reuters.com/article/us-health-coronavirus-handwashing-idUSKBN20S2N7. Accessed 25/4/2020.
9 For example, Gross, R.D. (2015). *Psychology;The Science of Mind and Behaviour* (7th ed.). London: Hodder Education.
10 Jahoda, M. (1958). Joint Commission on Mental Health and Illness Monograph Series: Vol. 1. Current Concepts of Positive Mental Health. *Basic Books*. https://doi.org/10.1037/11258-000.
11 Jahoda, M. (2009). *Employment and Unemployment: A Social-Psychological Analysis* (The Psychology of Social Issues). Cambridge: Cambridge University Press.
12 Maslow, A.H. (1987). *Motivation and Personality* (3rd ed.). London: Pearson Education.
13 Lindner, R. (1952, 1971). *The Revolutionist's Handbook*. New York: Grove Press, p. 4.
14 My paraphrase (not a direct quotation) from Dodge, R., Daly, A., Huyton, J. & Sanders, L. (2012). The Challenge of Defining Wellbeing. *International Journal of Wellbeing*, 2 (3), 222–235. doi:10.5502/ijw.v2i3.4. Accessed 3/5/2020.
15 Cox, T. (1975). The Nature and Management of Stress. *New Behaviour*, 25, pp. 493–495.

16 McCleod, S. (2010). Stress and Live Events. *Simply Psychology*. www.simplypsychology.org/SRRS.html. Accessed 28/4/2020. Take the Holmes and Rahe Stress Test at: www.mindtools.com/pages/article/newTCS_82.htm. Accessed 28/4/2020. Taking the test in the final week of writing this book, in lockdown, I scored 327!
17 Rahe, R.H. & Arthur, R.J. (1978). Life Change and Illness Studies: Past History and Future Directions. *Journal of Human Stress*, 4 (1), pp. 3–15.
18 Canadian Medical Hall of Fame (no date). Hans Selye, MD PhD. See: www.cdnmedhall.org/inductees/hansselye. Accessed 28/4/2020.
19 The term 'fight or flight' was coined by physiologist Walter Cannon in 1915.
20 American Psychological Association. (no date). See: www.apa.org/helpcenter/stress-body. Accessed 5/5/2020.
21 Wood, G.W. (2019). *Letters to a New Student. Tips to Study Smarter from a Psychologist*. London & New York: Routledge.
22 Given the Greek origins of each prefix, the two types of stress can be thought of as dystopian and utopian – loosely.
23 Yerkes, R.M. & Dodson, J.D. (1908). The Relation of Strength of Stimulus to Rapidity of Habit-formation. *Journal of Comparative Neurology and Psychology*, 18 (5), pp. 459–482.
24 Lazarus, R.S. & Folkman, S. (1984). *Stress, Appraisal and Coping*. New York: Springer, p. 19.
25 McLeod, S. (2015). Stress Management. *Simply Psychology*. See: www.simplypsychology.org/stress-management.html. Accessed 3/5/2020. And: Penley, J.A., Tomaka, J. & Wiebe, J.S. (2002). The Association of Coping to Physical and Psychological Health Outcomes: A Meta-analytic Review. *Journal of Behavioral Medicine*, 25 (6), pp. 551–603.
26 McLeod (2015). And: Penley et al. (2002).
27 Heid, M. (2018). You Asked: Is It Bad for You to Read the News Constantly? *Time*. See: https://time.com/5125894/is-reading-news-bad-for-you/ Accessed 9/5/2020.
28 Including Richard Lazarus.
29 Kanner, A.D., Coyne, J.C., Schaefer, C. & Lazarus, R.S. (1981). Comparison of Two Modes of Stress Measurement: Daily Hassles and Uplifts Versus Major Life Events. *Journal of Behavioral Medicine*, 4 (1), pp. 1–39.
30 Maddi, S. (2002). The Story of Hardiness: Twenty Years of Theorizing, Research & Practice. *Consulting Psychology Journal: Practice and Research*, 54 (3), pp. 173–185.
31 Wood, G.W. (2019). *Letters to a New Student. Tips to Study Smarter from a Psychologist*. London & New York: Routledge. The book is based on a series of brief, problem-page style letters that can be read in any order. It is based on three factors: *foundation*, *managing obstacles*, and *practical psychology*.
32 Katz, D. (1960) cited in Wood (2019). And: Berg, I.K. & Szabo, P. (2005). *Brief Coaching for Lasting Solutions*. London: W.W. Norton.
33 Selhub (2005), Pinilla (2008) and Lieberman (2013), all cited in Wood (2019).
34 Rhodes (2013) cited in Wood (2019).
35 Quan (2016), Alhola & Polo-Kantola (2007), and Gordon (2013), all cited in Wood (2019).
36 Jones & Gould (1996) cited in Wood (2019).
37 Watson (2015) and Lange (2013), both cited in Wood (2019).
38 Bryom (2016), Webb (2016), Lazarus & Folkman (1984), also cited in Wood (2019).

39 Kabat-Zinn (1994) cited in Bazin, O. & Kuyken, W. (2017). The Mindfulness Approach. Promises and Perils in the 21st Century. *Psychology Review*, November, pp. 20–23.
40 Wolpe (1991) cited in Wood (2019).
41 Hardy et al. (1996) cited in Wood (2019).
42 Bazin & Kuyken (2017), pp. 20–23.
43 Briers, S. (2012). *Psychobabble. Exploding the Myths of the self-Help Generation*. London: Pearson, p. 73.
44 Briers (2012).
45 Briers (2012), p. 73.
46 Luborsky et al. (1975) cited in Bergsma (2007). But originally: S. Rosenzweig (1936). Some Implicit Common Factors in Diverse Methods of Psychotherapy. *American Journal of Orthopsychiatry*, 6 (3), pp. 412–415. https://doi.org/10.1111/j.1939-0025.1936.tb05248.x.
47 Briers (2012).
48 Hubble & Miller (2004) cited in Bergsma (2007).
49 Talmon, M. (1990). *Single Session Therapy: Maximizing the Effect of the First (and Often Only) Therapeutic Encounter*. Chichester: Jossey-Bass.
50 See: https://twitter.com/matthaig1/status/1256982826978873344. Accessed 7/5/2020.
51 *BBC News* (2020). Coronavirus: Book Sales Surge as Readers Seek Escapism and Education. www.bbc.co.uk/news/entertainment-arts-52048582. Accessed 7/5/2020. Also: *The Telegraph* (2020). Reading 'Can Help Reduce Stress'. www.telegraph.co.uk/news/health/news/5070874/Reading-can-help-reduce-stress.html. Accessed 7/5/2020.
52 Family Links (no date). Emotional Health and Wellbeing – Good Mental Health Starts Here. See: www.familylinks.org.uk/post/emotional-health-and-wellbeing-good-mental-health-starts-here. Accessed 7/5/2020.

FURTHER READING

BOOKS

Andreski, S. (1972). *Social Science as Sorcery*. London: Andre Deutsch.

Armstrong, K. (2010). *Twelve Steps to a Compassionate Life*. Maine: Thorndike Windsor Paragon.

Briers, S. (2012). *Psychobabble. Exploding the Myths of the self-Help Generation*. London: Pearson.

Csikszentmihalyi, M. (1997). *Finding Flow: The Psychology of Engagement with Everyday Life*. New York: Perseus Books.

Ehrenreich, B. (2009). *Smile or Die: How Positive Thinking Fooled America & the World*. London: Granta.

Grenville Cleave, B. (2016). *Positive Psychology*. London: Icon Books.

Keyes, C.L.M. & Haidt, J. (2002). *Flourishing: Positive Psychology and the Life Well-Lived*. Washington: American Psychological Association.

Lilienfeld, S.O., Lynn, S.J., Ruscio, J. & Beyerstein, B.L. (2010). *50 Great Myths of Popular Psychology. Shattering Widespread Misconceptions about Human Behaviour*. Chichester: Wiley-Blackwell.

Lindner, R. (1971). *The Revolutionist's Handbook*. New York: Grove Press.
Rotenberg, K.J. (2018). *The Psychology of Trust*. London & New York: Routledge.
Salerno, S. (2005). *SHAM. How the Gurus of the Self-Help Movement Make Us Helpless*. London & Boston: Nicholas Brealey.
Seligman, M. (2011). *Flourish: A New Understanding of Happiness and Wellbeing: The Practical Guide to Using Positive Psychology to Make You Happier and Healthier*. London: Nicholas Brealey.
Watzlawick, P. (1993). *The Situation Is Hopeless, but Not Serious: The Pursuit of Unhappiness*. London: W.W. Norton & Company.
Wilkinson, R. & Pickett, K. (2009). *The Spirit Level: Why More Equal Societies Almost Always Do Better*. London: Allen Lane.
Wood, G.W. (2013). *Unlock Your Confidence*. London: Watkins Books.
Wood, G.W, (2018). *The Psychology of Gender*. London & New York: Routledge.
Wood, G.W. (2019). *Letters to a New Student. Tips to Study Smarter from a Psychologist*. London & New York: Routledge.

NOVELS

Inspirational

Illusions: The Adventures of a Reluctant Messiah by Richard Bach. Arrow Books, 2001.
Jonathan Livingston Seagull: A Story by Richard Bach. Harper Collins, 1994.
The Little Prince by Antoine de Saint-Exupéry (Kathryn Woods translation). Picador, 1982.

Dystopian

Nineteen Eighty-Four (1984) by George Orwell/ Penguin Modern Classics, 2004 (originally 1949).
Fahrenheit 451 by Ray Bradbury. Flamingo Modern Classics, 1999 (originally 1953).
Swastika Night by Katharine Burdekin. The Feminist Press, 1985 (Originally 1937).

FILMS

Big Fish (2003, directed by Tim Burton).
Life Is Beautiful (1999, directed by Roberto Benigni).
Pleasantville (1998, directed by Gary Ross).

WEBSITES

For a range of copyright free psychometric measures on subjective wellbeing visit: https://eddiener.com/scales

To discover your values and character strengths visit: www.viacharacter.org/

Read, affirm and share the 'Charter for Compassion': https://charterforcompassion.org/charter/affirm

To get in touch with the author to discuss coaching and research email: info@drgarywood.co.uk. Or visit: www.drgarywood.co.uk

3 Opportunities of technology to promote health and well-being

Saskia M. Kelders and Matthew Howard

This chapter was first published in *eHealth Research, Theory and Development* and cross-referencing relates to chapters in the original volume. Please visit www.routledge.com/9781138230439 for more information about the book

In this chapter, we will show why and how technology, in particular, Information and Communication Technology (ICT), is a very appropriate way to promote health and well-being. This is further explained by briefly going into the evolution of technologies within the domain of eHealth. We exemplify the opportunities of technology by going more into depth with four examples: cognitive computing, embodied conversational agents, virtual and augmented reality, and wearable technology for self-tracking. You will see that many technologies are 'smart' and use a form of artificial intelligence (AI). We will introduce some building blocks for these smart technologies: machine learning, natural language processing, image recognition and neural networks. Lastly, we will describe different software development models to give insight into the process that leads to these kinds of technologies. After completing this chapter, you will be able to:

- explain the advantages of technology for health and knows what possibilities of technology induce these advantages.
- discuss the evolution of technology, in particular technologies relating to eHealth.
- discuss different examples of technologies and their opportunities for health and well-being.
- explain the basics of common building blocks of technology, namely, machine learning, natural language processing, image recognition and neural networks.
- name and explain different software design models.

Advantages of technology for health

Healthcare and technology always have had a complicated relationship: on the one hand, technology has the possibility to make healthcare more effective and efficient. For example, many early technologies, such as the microscope, have been used to gain more insight into our own health. On the other hand, technologies and innovation in general, have been notoriously slow to disseminate in healthcare (Berwick, 2003). Benefits have been seen from introducing innovations and technology–from bringing fruit on ships to overcome scurvy in the 1500s to the implementation of electronic health records in many countries in recent decades–but actual implementation has often been slow and difficult. Later in this chapter, and in this book, we will go into more depth about these implementation issues (see Chapter 12). But first, let's look at the advantages of technology for health, well-being and healthcare.

A specific form of technology that has received a lot of attention in the healthcare domain, is the Internet. From the rise of the Internet, research into using this technology to improve health and healthcare has been increasing rapidly. Eysenbach's seminal 2001 paper 'What is eHealth?' names 10 e's that characterize what eHealth should be about (Eysenbach, 2001). These e's range from efficiency and enhancing quality to empowerment and equity: all advantages that using technology as computers and networks should bring. A systematic review in 2006 showed that reasons for delivering health interventions of the Internet, according to the researchers, were reducing costs (for users and healthcare), increasing convenience, reducing stigma, being able to provide information on time and increased user and supplier control of the intervention (Griffiths, Lindenmeyer, Powell, Lowe, & Thorogood, 2006). Many of these expected advantages are still applicable today, as was discussed in Chapter 1. But why is technology (in this case the Internet) able to provide these advantages?

Technology as a persuader

An answer to this question can be found in the reasons that Fogg gives why computer persuaders can sometimes be better than human persuaders at influencing attitudes and behaviour (Fogg, 2002):

Technology is more persistent than human beings

After a while, humans will get tired of trying to persuade someone. Technology, of course, does not have this fatigue, as it can continue to persuade its end users indefinitely. Of course, this also raises an ethical issue. If the technology doesn't automatically stop trying to persuade after a while, the developers should probably build in a stop function.

Technology offers greater anonymity

When talking to a human persuader, it is difficult, if not impossible, to stay anonymous. With technology, this is easier. Many online behaviour change programmes offer the possibility to sign up anonymously, which can be a huge advantage for sensitive subjects like psychological problems or substance abuse.

Technology can manage huge volumes of data

Humans can process a lot of data, but when it comes to managing huge volumes of data (Big Data), technology has a clear advantage. This can give technology more persuasive power, because technology can back up a certain message with the data that supports it.

Technology uses many modalities to influence

Technology can present information in many different ways, including text, audio and video. Because of this, technology can match each person's individual preferences to the persuasive methods it uses.

Technology is scalable

This may be the largest and most practical advantage. People can only reach a limited number of other people. But by using technology, many more people can be reached without a large increase in cost. Especially in public health, this is a major advantage, and this is the argument that is most often used for delivering a behaviour change programme by means of technology.

Technology can go where humans cannot go or may not be welcome

Technology can be, and is, everywhere! Even in places that you wouldn't allow a human persuader to be. We know that for many behaviour change techniques to be effective, timing is important. For example, consider changing your tooth-brushing behaviour. Having the dentist telling you how to brush your teeth may be persuasive when you are in the dental chair, but chances are you will have forgotten about it when you are at home and ready to brush your teeth. But technology, like a smart toothbrush, can persuade you to continue brushing your teeth for a while longer that night in your own bathroom. Imagine the dentist doing that!

This list of why computers can be persuasive brings us closer to some of the specific opportunities of technology that we may be able to harness to improve health and healthcare. In many sensitive healthcare areas, the anonymity that technology can offer may be one of the largest opportunities. The ability of technology to manage huge volumes of data and to 'do' things with the data seems to be one of the advantages that comes into play when dealing with, for instance, electronic patient records, but also with the rise of 'big data'. Scaling easily, so reaching more people, is especially important in delivering public health interventions to people at risk, for example, to smokers or to people who are overweight. It is impossible to reach all of these people with human caregivers, while technology gives us the scalability that is needed for this. Another advantage of computer persuaders that is extremely relevant for health and well-being is that technology can intervene at the right time and at the appropriate place (IJsselsteijn, de Kort, Midden, Eggen, & van den Hoven, 2006). By using, for example, sensor technologies, it is possible to gain information about the context of a person and by using algorithms (to manage all this data), this information can be used to select the right time and place to, for example, deliver a persuasive health-related message. Because the latest technology is something you always have with you (e.g. smartphones and wearables), the persuasion becomes independent of time and place. And this is something that human persuaders have not been able to achieve.

But how did technology gain all these advantages? Or were they there all the time? In the next section, we will go deeper into the evolution of technology to show where these advantages came from.

The evolution of eHealth technologies

As stated before, the Internet caused a huge rise in the use of technology for health purposes, but the rise of the Internet was not the only cause for the increasing interest in using technology for health. In this section, we will give a short overview of important technological developments that have had an influence on healthcare.

Types of technologies

Figure 3.1 presents a timeline which indicates when some 'older' medical technologies were introduced and shows several aspects of the rise of the Internet, smartphones and wearables. It is important to note first that this timeline is by no means exhaustive: there are many more technologies and events that have had an impact on health and healthcare. Figure 3.1 is merely meant to give an idea of the kind of technologies and the pace of innovation. Second, it is important to differentiate between medical technology, for example, the X-ray and the MRI, and eHealth technologies, for example, the Fitbit, web-based interventions and apps on a smartphone. Figure 3.1 shows both types of technology, medical and eHealth,

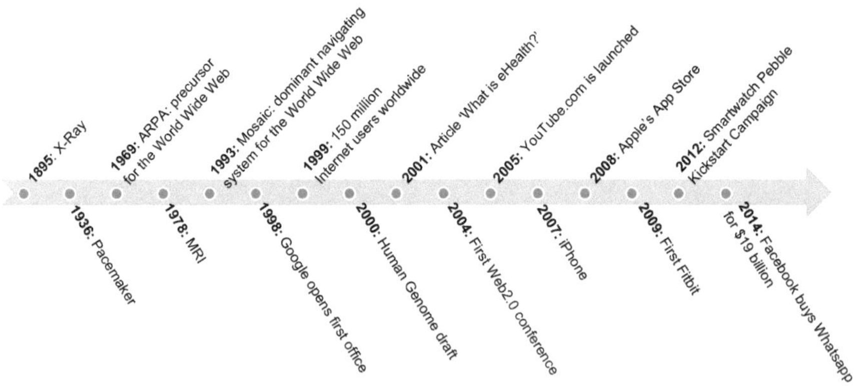

Figure 3.1 Timeline with examples of medical and eHealth-related technologies and events

to illustrate the breadth of technology used in healthcare, but the focus of this chapter is on eHealth technologies, which is mainly Information and Communication Technology (ICT).

What becomes clear from this timeline is that the pace of innovation, especially in the Internet area, is very fast. This is often called the '*digital revolution*': the very fast and impactful changes brought about by digital computing and communication technology. Mosaic, one of the early Web browsers which made the World Wide Web popular, was only introduced in 1993! Nowadays, it seems like the Internet, and easy ways to access it, have always been there. The way that the Internet is used also changes very fast. In the early days, the Internet was more of a read-only platform, with only a relatively few people creating content and many people acting merely as consumers of content. Nowadays, everybody can, and does, create content with social media, such as Facebook, but this so-called *Web 2.0* has only been around from about 2004.

Figure 3.2 presents a more in-depth overview of the evolution of *persuasive technologies* (e.g. technologies that are designed to change the behaviour or attitudes of people, see Chapter 11) in the context of health (Chatterjee & Price, 2009). This figure shows that eHealth technologies have evolved from prescriptive systems, via descriptive systems, to environmental and automated systems. The early prescriptive systems involved fundamentally human, static one-on-one persuasion where healthcare providers used technology as telephones and CD-ROMs that could be given to patients for extra information.

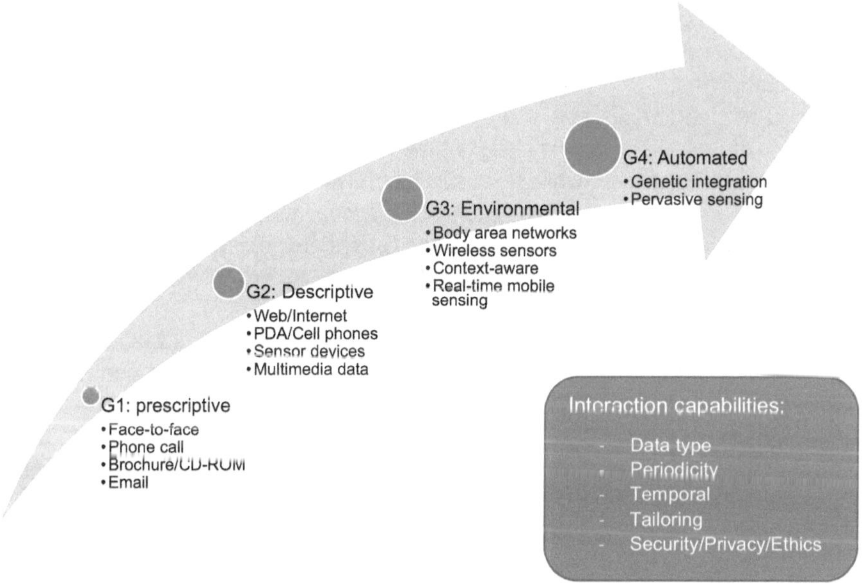

Figure 3.2 Roadmap of evolution of persuasive technologies

Source: Adapted from Chatterjee and Price (2009)

There was no real interaction with the system or technology itself. The second generation technologies, descriptive systems, were mainly web-based systems where text and later multimedia information was shared with and among users. The use of sensors started in the second generation, but evolved in the third generation, where the data from sensors and other context-aware technologies are used to learn about the current state of the user of the technology (monitoring) so that 'just-in-time' persuasive messages can be given to influence behaviour (coaching). The latest generation of persuasive systems is characterized by more pervasive sensing and the use of smart algorithms to automatically personalize feedback and support, making human intervention minimal or not needed anymore.

Human, technological and interaction foundations

As can been seen in Figure 3.2, this evolution did not come out of nowhere, but was built on three other layers: human elements, technological foundations and interaction capabilities. The human elements layer shows that it is always important to keep in mind that the actual use of technology by a person is a form of behaviour. To understand this behaviour, it is important to know about, for instance, behaviour change theories and psychology. We have already touched upon the technological foundations in the timeline in Figure 3.1. Without these foundations, there could be no evolution of eHealth technologies. The third layer shows the interaction capabilities that are important and were necessary to bring about the different generations of eHealth technology:

- Data type: first generation systems (G1) mainly used text as their data type, as newer generation systems use more data types as audio, video and sensor information.
- Periodicity: earlier systems had a low periodicity of exchange with a low frequency of updates of content (e.g. a new version of a CD-ROM only appeared after months or years), while later systems have a much higher frequency of updates (from weekly updates of content to a website with health information, to daily and continuous updates in G3 and G4 systems that provide just-in-time and personalized coaching messages).
- Temporal: the way time is measured and used also differs. Earlier systems measure time in discrete units as years, months or days, while the later generations of systems work in real time, so time becomes a more continuous measure.
- *Tailoring*: earlier generation systems hardly provided any tailoring, and information was the same for all users, while later generation systems use data to be able to provide the most appropriate content to the right user, with a very high level of tailoring, called customization in the original model (Chatterjee & Price, 2009).
- Security/privacy/ethics: all of these capabilities have their own security, privacy and ethical issues which need to be addressed in order to make the most out of the opportunities that exist.

The fact that many technologies we rely on and that seem to have always been there are relatively new also has an impact on eHealth research and interventions. First, research has not fully explored the possibilities of existing technology. There has just not been enough time to fully explore everything that is possible. The pace of technological change has been so fast that research struggles to keep up with it (Patrick et al., 2016). For example, within mental health interventions, lately there has been a shift from web-based interventions to apps/mobile interventions, which fits with recent trends in technology. However, there are still many opportunities within web-based interventions (e.g. in-depth *tailoring*, use of multimedia) that have not yet been fully studied. Second, research has not fully explored and understood how people use technology and what influence it has on us. We know that using technology has an impact on our attitudes and behaviour, but exactly how and in what ways is not fully known. This makes it difficult to predict what the (long-term) influence is of, for example, always being able to monitor your own health, and the possible negative consequences of technology that aims to influence behaviour. We should in keep in mind that technology is not necessarily the solution: there are many cases where technology is not needed and where it will not have added value. Together this shows that, for eHealth researchers and developers, it may not always be necessary to jump to the newest available technology. There are so many opportunities of already existing technologies that have not yet been tapped into that trying them may well be a worthwhile endeavour. We might also need some time to evaluate and reflect on the impact technology has had on us, and how it has changed our daily lives. This understanding can help us find new ways of promoting health and well-being by making smart use of (existing) technologies in the best possible way.

Examples of technology for health and healthcare

To give some more in-depth information about the opportunities of technology for health, we discuss four different technologies that have a lot of potential for health, well-being and healthcare. These examples show how the development of technology influences its potential for health. Furthermore, these technologies illustrate the importance for each member of an eHealth development team to have some knowledge of the technology that is being used in order to be able to understand and optimally make use of the possibilities of the technology (also see Chapter 7).

Cognitive computing

A *'cognitive computer'* can be described as a system that mimics but does not replicate the functioning of the human brain, they therefore complement rather than replace human cognition. One example of this type of technology is IBM's 'Watson'. Watson first rose to prominence when it was a contestant on the quiz show *Jeopardy* in the United States. In *Jeopardy*, the contestants are given general knowledge clues in the form of answers in order to determine the question being asked. In 2011, Watson was able to win the quiz against champion players (videos of the encounter can be found on YouTube). Key to this success was Watson's ability to ingest large volumes of broad unstructured information/data and answer questions posed in natural language against this information through a process known as *Deep Question Answering* (DeepQA). Such open domain deep QA is considered highly challenging, requiring a synthesis of information retrieval, *natural language processing*, knowledge representation and reasoning, *machine learning* and computer-human interfaces (Ferrucci et al., 2010).

The ability to 'train' a system such as Watson using a combination of structured and unstructured data has significant potential for healthcare. This is the case for 'Clinical Decision Support Systems' or 'Expert systems' in particular, which can provide support to healthcare practitioners, for example, in the provision of patient treatment recommendations. In this case, cognitive technologies can support the synthesis and interpretation of information, for example, patient longitudinal data, and analyze such patient data against the 'corpus' (e.g. data set) that the system has been trained with. In principle, such systems have the potential to be completely unbiased in terms of how the patient data is interpreted and unconstrained in the amount of information they can draw on, provided that the underlying training data and approach is unbiased itself. These technologies can, for example, generate treatment recommendations that can be reviewed and considered by the treating physician. In addition to decision support, the use of such technologies to generate an instantaneous second opinion for a patient, without the need to see a further physician, is also being explored. Another possible avenue is the ability to improve adherence to treatment guidelines by healthcare professionals. It should be stressed, however, that these are supportive technologies designed to help guide treatment decisions but not to replace the patient-physician paradigm.

A clinical version of Watson has been developed and is known as 'Watson for Oncology'. This was developed in partnership with a US clinical site, Memorial Sloan Kettering. This system was trained using a range of sources, including best-practice treatment guidelines, the scientific literature, clinical trial reports and several thousand hours of clinical time to test and refine the technology and training. The system ingests a patient record and makes treatment recommendations based on its training, in this case, across breast, colorectal and lung cancers. Watson for Oncology is now being deployed at clinical sites across the world. Early data presented at the San Antonio Breast Cancer Symposium in 2016 suggests a high degree of concordance between physician recommendations and those of the platform (Somashekhar et al., 2017), although more studies will be required to demonstrate the effectiveness of such technologies and their impact.

While there is significant potential for such systems, effective governance is critical. Clinical oversight is crucial, and new releases of the system must be robustly technically and clinically validated prior to use. Testing of machine learning must be performed in a controlled fashion to prevent contamination of the original training material. Moreover, critical to the success of technologies such as artificial intelligence is the ability to understand what has led to a given recommendation being made, for example, a chemotherapy treatment algorithm. This is especially important given that a machine learning model can be difficult to decompose. As a result, a system must always present the underlying evidence base (e.g. publication or clinical trial) that has led the cognitive computer to arrive at a particular recommendation based on the particular patient record.

Embodied conversational agents

In many health interventions, users benefit from receiving support. For example, we know from research that guided online interventions for people with depressive symptoms, where a counsellor sends (often weekly) feedback messages to the client, are more effective than unguided versions (Andersson & Cuijpers, 2009). Also, when trying to change your health behaviour, we know it is beneficial to get feedback that is tailored to you and your situation (Noar, Benac, & Harris, 2007). However, much is unknown about what kind of support is needed within health interventions and from whom the support needs to come. For example, within the context of eHealth for mental issues, studies have shown that task-related support (e.g. 'Thank you for submitting your homework. It was well on time!') can be enough to increase adherence and effectiveness of these interventions (Talbot, 2012). However, users often do express a need for some form of emotional support (Scholten, Kelders, & van Gemert-Pijnen, 2017). Interestingly, it seems like both forms of support do not need to come from a care provider like a psychologist but can also be given by lay persons, or even be automated (Kelders, Bohlmeijer, Pots, & van Gemert-Pijnen, 2015; Talbot, 2012).

Embodied conversational agents (ECAs) seem to be able to provide this support. An ECA can be described as an animated computer character that simulates face-to-face conversation using, for example, voice, hand gesture, gaze cues, and other nonverbal behaviour (Cassell, Bickmore, Campbell, Vilhjálmsson, & Yan, 2000). Figure 3.3 shows Laura, one of the early ECAs in the healthcare context. Research has shown that users of an intervention to increase physical activity supported by Laura did form a relationship with her that they found helpful. In this case, however, it did not result in significantly better improvement in physical activity (Bickmore & Picard, 2005).

The way that ECAs build this relationship with users is by engaging in conversations. This can be done in a relatively simple way by, for example, having the user select a response from a list of predefined messages and build in algorithms that specify what message the ECA should give in return. This way the conversation is performed in written text that can be spoken aloud by the agent in a structured form. The agent can further stimulate the conversation by expressing some form of empathy, for example, showing interest or understanding by showing 2D images of the agent expressing a certain emotion at a certain time (Bickmore & Picard, 2005). On the other side of the spectrum, the conversation can also be held in a technically more complex way, for example, by having the user actually talk to the agent and having the agent interpret the spoken text and formulate an appropriate response. The agent can be depicted as a 3D virtual character that moves and expresses emotions in real time. This way, the conversation is much more versatile but also much more technically complex. Not only does the agent need to be able to interpret spoken text but this text can

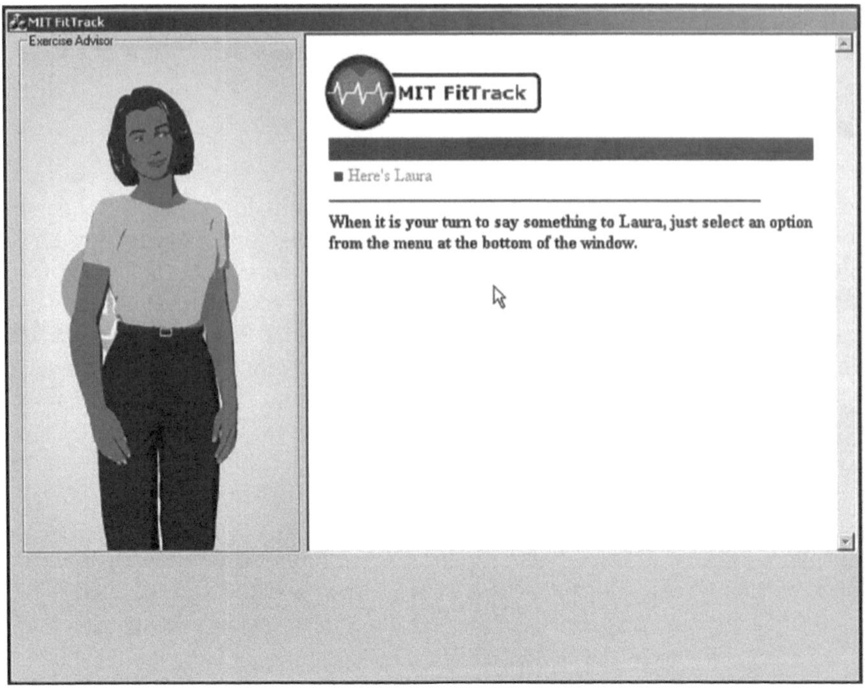

Figure 3.3 ECA Laura in the MIT FitTrack intervention

Source: From http://affect.media.mit.edu/projectpages/relational/

be virtually about anything, meaning that there needs to be more advanced AI methods to create an appropriate response (Cassell, 2001). Furthermore, more complex ECAs try to not only react to the user, but also proactively give support when they sense the user needs this. This can, for instance, be done through measuring and trying to alleviate frustration using artificial intelligence methods (Klein, Moon, & Picard, 2002).

Based on the complexity of ECAs, a distinction can be made between responsive and non-responsive agents, whereby the first is the most complex version. Although responsive agents seem to hold the most potential for eHealth technology, these responsive agents also show the largest 'risks'. As it is very complex to always react appropriately at the right time, mistakes are often made, resulting in users disengaging from the conversation and/or reducing their trust in the agent. At the moment, very promising results are shown with these agents, but only in short timespans (only one or a few sessions) and in experimental environments instead of for longer period of times in the daily life of people who need to be supported with their health behaviour. It might well be that in some contexts, for example, self-guided online interventions, simpler non-responsive agents might be enough to support users.

Virtual reality

The popularity of virtual reality has dramatically increased recently: it is frequently being used by the gaming industry, in advertising, real estate and healthcare. *Virtual reality* (VR) is an advanced form of a human-computer interface that enables the user to interact with and be immersed in a computer-generated environment (Schultheis & Rizzo, 2001). A couple of years ago, one could only use VR via expensive glasses that were hard to come by for consumers, but nowadays VR can be used via relatively cheap goggles that can be bought in regular shops. In line with its popularity in practice, many articles about the use of VR to improve (mental) health have been published recently. They focus, for example, on using VR to reduce pain, train relaxation skills, eliminate fear of heights or even assess sexual preferences of paedophiles.

It might seem that VR is a new, state-of-the-art technology, but it actually has been around for a while. The first studies about VR in mental healthcare were published over 20 years ago, for example, a study on fear of flying (Rothbaum, Hodges, Watson, Kessler, & Opdyke, 1996). At first, VR mainly focused on the treatment of phobias, since it can be used to expose patients to specific, fear-eliciting stimuli (Diemer, Alpers, Peperkorn, Shiban, & Mühlberger, 2015). It has also been found to be effective in the treatment of other psychiatric disorders such as autism, obsessive-compulsive disorder, attention deficit disorders and post-traumatic stress disorder (North & North, 2016; Turner & Casey, 2014). Many of these studies have pointed out the potential of VR: a meta-analysis on VR in psychological interventions showed that VR interventions are very effective when compared to control groups without interventions, and moderately effective when compared to control groups with another intervention (Turner & Casey, 2014). Despite these positive results, VR was not a popular topic of research and was hardly used in practice. A main reason for its recent popularity is the availability of consumer VR glasses, which has made it an accessible, well-known technology.

A specific characteristic of VR that appeals to researchers and practitioners is its ability to 'immerse' the user in a simulated environment (Diemer et al., 2015), which cannot be reached in face-to-face contact. *Immersion* positively influences a feeling of presence in the user, which represents the extent to which a user has the feeling of actually being in a VR environment (Botella et al., 2009). If a person experiences this presence, real emotions can be activated, which means that specific skills (e.g. coping strategies) can be assessed and trained in realistic environments (Price, Mehta, Tone, & Anderson, 2011; Tichon & Mavin, 2016). There are several ways to reach this feeling of presence, for example, via 360° videos of real-life environments such as dolphins swimming in the ocean, or animations created by developers that can represent personally relevant environments and persons, such as your local bar where you can interact with an avatar that resembles your mother-in-law. In some cases, other modalities such as smell or touch are used to increase the realism. This adaptability of VR can enable tailoring to the needs and skills of patients.

The possibilities of VR for healthcare depend on the characteristics of technology, so new technological developments will impact research on and use of VR in practice. For example, interaction with VR avatars is currently either non-present or simulated via a microphone that transforms the voice of a therapist or coach, but developments in artificial intelligence can enable automated interaction. The emergence of other comparable types of technologies such as *augmented reality* can impact VR as well. Also, new technologies can be combined with VR: wearables that measure physiological states of users are used to provide insight into their reactions on VR scenarios.

Wearable technology for self-tracking

New advances in technology have resulted in numerous *wearable technologies for self-tracking*: technologies that are small enough to take with you, that are embedded into clothing or accessories, that measure information from your body and life. Examples are activity trackers and smartwatches. Devices such as these can measure, among other things, heartrate (variability), physical activity, sleep and body temperature (Figure 3.4). Often this information is not measured in isolation but accompanied by contextual information such as your location, what you are

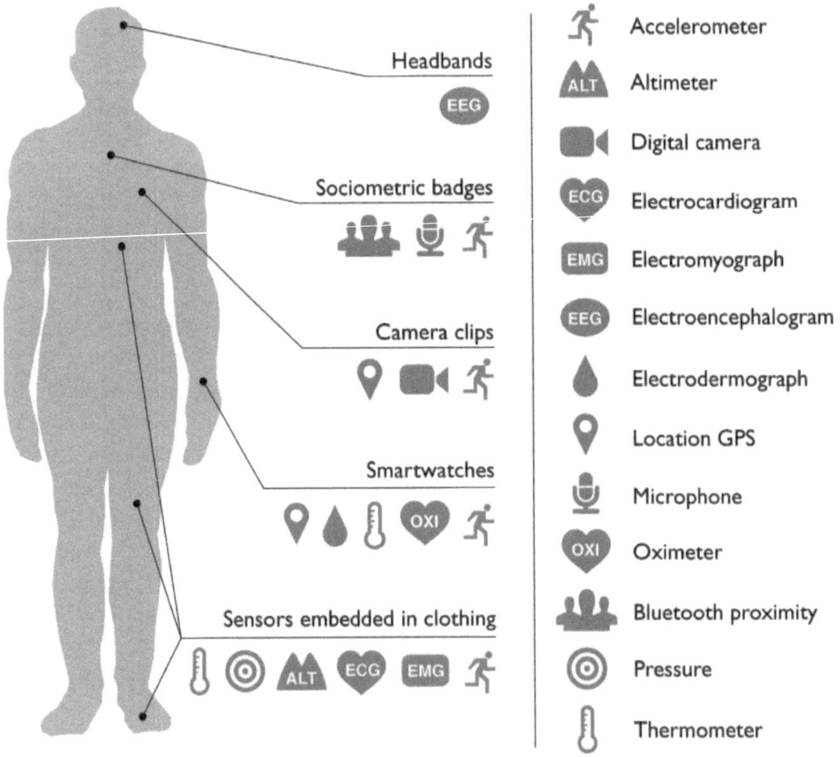

Figure 3.4 What can be measured

Source: Piwek et al. (2016)

doing (e.g. measured using experience sampling techniques) and the weather. As many of these devices are connected with your smartphone, the smartphone is often used to get this contextual information. Goals of these wearable technologies are not only to help the user get insight into their health and well-being but also to impact these in a positive way (Lentferink et al., 2017; Piwek, Ellis, Andrews, & Joinson, 2016).

Self-tracking technologies provide important opportunities that might assist in promoting healthy behaviour in large groups of people. First, these technologies provide objective data: they do not rely on questionnaires or other ways of self-reporting, which might bias the data, but use the actual real-time data that is gathered by sensors (Swan, 2013). Furthermore, in principle, the data is collected without input from the user, so it requires no effort and cannot be forgotten. Second, self-tracking technologies are widely available: many of these technologies are commercial, such as the Fitbit or the Apple Watch. This means that many people have access to these technologies without the need for them to be prescribed by, for instance, a care provider or researcher. This wide availability makes the potential group of people using these technologies very large. Lastly, self-tracking technologies have the opportunity to provide personal feedback: because of the objective, individual data, it is possible to provide feedback and advice that is tailored to the individual. By comparing the current values with the goals that a user has set, the technology can alert the user that he or she is not reaching his or her goal but also assist the user in reaching the goal by automatically analyzing the data to, for example, find the reason why he or she is not reaching his or her goal or to remind the user what successfully resolved the problem previously (Li, Dey, & Forlizzi, 2011).

However, at the moment, wearable technologies have not been shown to be really successful in actually promoting healthy behaviour (Patel, Asch, & Volpp, 2015; Piwek et al., 2016). It seems like the opportunities of self-tracking technology are also the reasons why these have not been very successful so far. First, the used sensors are not always validated for what they are supposed to measure, and large variations in accuracy have been observed between devices (Lee, Kim, & Welk, 2014). Furthermore, privacy remains an issue. With commercial self-tracking devices, the users often do not 'own' their data. It is stored by the manufacturer of the device who might sell the data to third parties. Although it is often said that only anonymized data is sold, this anonymization is often not good enough, so this data might be traced back to an individual (De Montjoye, Hidalgo, Verleysen, & Blondel, 2013). Second, although wearable devices are widely available, they are often used by the people who need them the least: younger people who are already quite healthy (Piwek et al., 2016). Moreover, many people don't use these devices for very long: after six months, 32% stop using them and even 50% do so after a year (Ledger & McCaffrey, 2014). Long-term engagement is an issue, possibly because the devices are not that good yet at providing personal feedback. At the moment, many devices only present data (e.g. current steps) but do not support the users' reflection about this data or assist the user in changing behaviour (Li et al., 2011). There is a need for smarter technology to automatically analyze the data to see patterns and to help the user answer the questions they might have about their data. This might be done by employing artificial intelligence.

Selected building blocks of technology used in eHealth

In all the technology examples of previous sections, technology is not a static tool but something that is smart in a way: it mimics the human brain and can understand and answer questions, it can engage in conversations and provide support, it provides a virtual environment where people can interact or it collects data and analyzes it to give personal feedback. All this can be seen as a form of artificial intelligence (AI). AI has recently come to prominence, driven by rapidly increasing levels of computational power combined with the availability of very large data sets that can be used to 'train' such systems. The term AI itself is broad and can be applied to a wide range of technologies. Indeed, Kris Hammond of Northwestern University describes AI in the following way: 'any program can be considered AI if it does something that we would normally think of as intelligent in humans'. This can be, for example, recognizing what is on a certain picture, or making a prediction of whether a participant will benefit from using a particular eHealth intervention. Some of the key technologies that underpin AI use cases in healthcare are machine learning, natural language processing, image recognition and neural networks. When understanding (new) eHealth technology and its possibilities, it is very beneficial to have a grasp of these building blocks.

Machine learning

Machine learning (ML) is a widely used computer science technology that has broad application to the healthcare space. Put simply, ML gives computers the ability to learn without being explicitly programmed (Munoz, 2014). Such learning can be considered 'supervised' when performed using labelled or annotated datasets, where each case is labelled with the outcome of interest (e.g. 'effective' or 'not effective' when predicting whether a certain treatment is effective for individual cases). Machine learning can also be unsupervised, where the training data is unlabelled. In practice, this means running multiple training cycles to improve computer algorithms using the labelled data before running unsupervised cycles to enhance the capability of the technology. Machine learning underpins platforms such as IBM Watson and Google Deepmind Health but can also be used to predict, for example, depressive symptoms by using phone data (e.g. GPS) (Canzian & Musolesi, 2015).

Natural language processing

Natural language processing (NLP) allows computers to process unstructured data such as machine readable text and effectively facilitates the connection between human language and machine perception. NLP has been in development since the 1950s, but it has been accelerating in capability since the 1980s through combination with machine learning techniques. The key to NLP is a process known as 'parsing', which is the analysis of a natural language sentence/block into component parts and the understanding of context and negation, for example, that 'no history of arrhythmia' is fundamentally different to 'long history of arrhythmia'. NLP allows data sources that previously had been inaccessible to technology-based approaches to become usable, such as patient medical records. IBM Watson makes extensive use of NLP to both ingest medical records and to process unstructured data sources such as treatment guidelines or literature publications, making this data a valuable source of information to use in, for example, machine learning algorithms or neural networks.

Image recognition

Rapid advances in computational vision are opening a broad range of applications. In healthcare, image recognition is often used in combination with technologies such as pattern recognition and machine learning (see above). This allows the development of technologies such as automated screening platforms for use in diagnostics of, for example, MRI images. While such technologies have been available for some time, the ability to combine image and pattern recognition with machine learning and other cognitive techniques is opening up a wide range of novel applications that have the potential to have significant impact in areas that often have limited resources, for example, radiology and pathology.

Neural networks

An artificial *neural network* is a computational approach that is based on the cellular architecture of the brain, with individual nodes (analogous to neurons) arranged in multiple layers. Such networks can be trained used techniques such as deep learning to perform certain functions. Many advanced AI approaches are based on the use of such neural networks, including image and speech recognition.

Google's Deepmind technology is a neural network-based technology with the goal to 'solve intelligence'. Such approaches are able to learn from experience and reinforcement learning. Deepmind Health is currently exploring the use of such approaches in a range of projects with the UK National Health Service, including applications in acute kidney injury and diabetic retinopathy.

Development of technology

In the previous sections, you have seen some examples of technologies that can be useful for eHealth, and you have gained a basic understanding of some of the underlying features. However, it is also important to get a grasp of how these technologies may be developed. This section will give an overview of a few well-known and much-used software development models, for example, the Waterfall and Spiral models, Agile and Scrum.

Waterfall and spiral design models

The *Waterfall Model of System Development* (Figure 3.5) is one of the earliest software development models. It is essentially a sequential model: once a phase is finished, you move on to the next phase. The process starts with requirements specification, moves on to designing, implementing (coding), verification (testing) and finally maintenance. Although this model is often used for large projects, it has received a lot of criticism, mainly because of the rigid nature of a sequential model: no changes are possible later because the requirements are finalized in the first stage and because testing is done at a late stage, it is harder to fix possible issues (Petersen, Wohlin, & Baca, 2009). Because of this, adaptations to the Waterfall model have been proposed (e.g. adding feedback loops between the phases), leading, for example, to the *Spiral design model* (Boehm, 1988). The Spiral model is also a sequential model, but it involves iterative cycles of the sequential phases. This way the model can cope with more complex projects where not all the requirements are known in advance, or where the requirements may change due to feedback on prototypes or new insights. The Waterfall and Spiral models are more traditional methods of software development and are used less and less in current practice.

Agile software development and Scrum

In 2001, different software development practitioners shared their view on what software development should be like in the 'Manifesto for *agile software development*' (Beck et al., 2001). Since then, numerous methods and practices have surfaced that share the values and principles stated in this manifesto. Agile development focuses on fast development of small pieces of software, making the approach

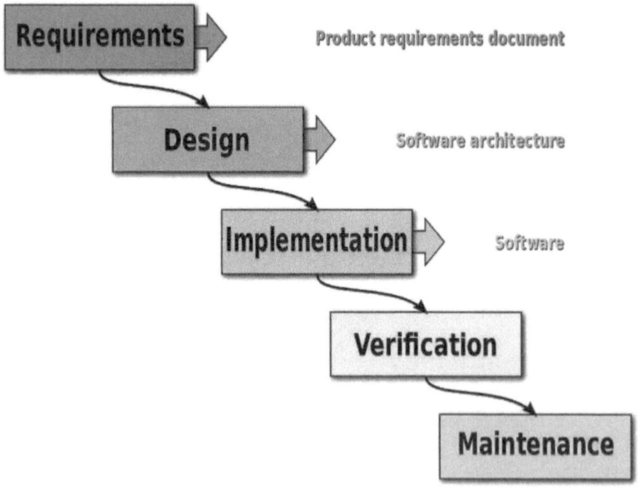

Figure 3.5 The Waterfall Model of System Development

Source: © Peter Kemp/Adapted from Paul Smith's work at Wikipedia more adaptive and able to deal with change. Core values are collaborative development, a 'lean' mentality where unnecessary work is minimized, more stakeholder involvement occurs in shaping and guiding the software and developers accept uncertainty, which encourages rapid and flexible response to change (Dingsøyr, Nerur, Balijepally, & Moe, 2012). One of the most widely used agile development frameworks is *Scrum*. In Scrum, developers work in teams of around three to nine people and break up their work in short cycles, called sprints. The work that needs to be done is collected in the product 'backlog': a list of everything that might be needed in the product. A few notable activities (e.g. 'events') are (Figure 3.6):

- sprint: a period of one month or less (often two weeks) in which a usable and potentially releasable product (increment) is developed. During a sprint, no changes are made that endanger the sprint goal, and the quality goals may not be decreased. However, the scope may be clarified or renegotiated when new insights are learned.
- sprint planning: a longer meeting (maximum eight hours) of the Scrum team to set the sprint goal and to determine how the needed work can be achieved.
- daily scrum: a short meeting (fifteen minutes) of the development team at the beginning of the day to check whether they are still on their way to achieve the sprint goals and to synchronize the activities of the day.

Agile approaches to technology development like Scrum are increasingly considered to be appropriate for the development of eHealth technology. The reasons for this are the often complex context that the technology needs to fit in, the large number of different stakeholders and the difficulty of specifying each requirement for the technology in advance. Moreover, more recently, there has been a call not only to apply these principles in the development of eHealth technology but also to use them in the way research into eHealth technology is conducted and disseminated (Hekler et al., 2016).

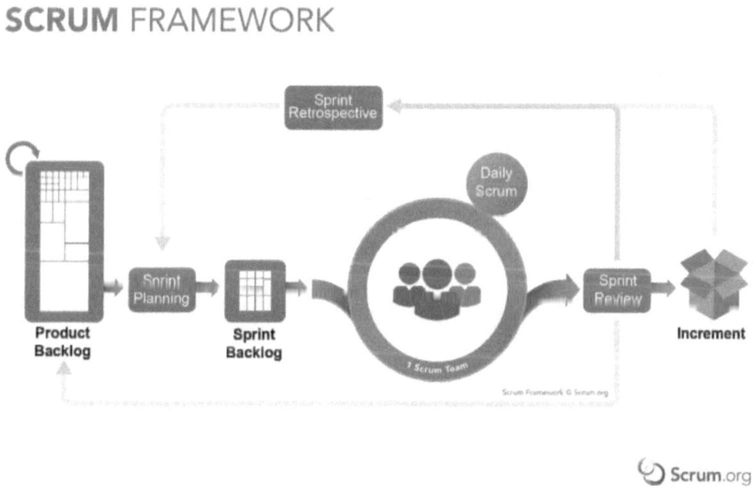

Figure 3.6 Scrum framework

Conclusion

In this chapter, you have seen that technology offers many opportunities to improve health and well-being. Characteristics of technology as persistence and being able to deal with large amounts of data can make technology an effective persuader. We have seen that the pace of innovation in technology is very fast. This makes it difficult, if not impossible, for researchers and practitioners in related fields to keep up to date with the latest technology. However, it is important for everyone in the field of eHealth to have some knowledge of what technology can do. One of the things technology can do is be 'smart', using artificial intelligence, and this chapter has given an introduction to the building blocks of AI. Combined with the basic knowledge of the software development process, these insights can help you in finding the added value of technology for your specific goal and in working with the software developers who might be able to develop the technology with you. The take-home messages for this chapter are:

- Technology offers specific opportunities to be an influential persuader with its persistence, anonymity, ability to deal with large amounts of data, use of many modalities, its scalability and its being able to be everywhere.
- The pace of technological innovation has been very fast in the past and is expected to stay fast.
- Cognitive computing, embodied conversational agents, virtual reality and wearable devices for self-tracking are examples of useful technologies to improve health and well-being.
- Many technologies are, or need to be, smart, and this can be achieved by using AI.
- Machine learning, natural language processing, image recognition and neural networks are building blocks underlying AI.
- Waterfall and Spiral models are traditional software development models that are more or less sequential and have trouble with the unpredictability of the development process. Agile software development, such as Scrum, is much more flexible and able to deal with change, making it more suitable for the development of eHealth technologies.

Key references for further reading

Cassell, J. (2001). Embodied conversational agents: Representation and intelligence in user interfaces. *AI Magazine*, *22*(4), 67.

Dingsøyr, T., Nerur, S., Balijepally, V., & Moe, N. B. (2012). A decade of agile methodologies: Towards explaining agile software development. *Journal of Systems and Software*, *85*(6), 1213–1221.

Ferrucci, D., Brown, E., Chu-Carroll, J., Fan, J., Gondek, D., Kalyanpur, A. A., . . . & Prager, J. (2010). Building Watson: An overview of the DeepQA project. *AI Magazine*, *31*(3), 59–79.

Li, I., Dey, A. K., & Forlizzi, J. (2011). Understanding my data, myself: Supporting self-reflection with ubicomp technologies. In *Proceedings of the 13th international conference on ubiquitous computing*.

Munoz, A. (2014). *Machine learning and optimization*. Retrieved on March 2, 2016 from www.cims.nyu.edu/~ munoz/files/ml_optimization.pdf [WebCite Cache ID 6fiLfZvnG].

References

Andersson, G., & Cuijpers, P. (2009). Internet-based and other computerized psychological treatments for adult depression: A meta-analysis. *Cognitive Behaviour Therapy*, *38*(4), 196–205.

Beck, K., Beedle, M., van Bennekum, A., Cockburn, A., Cunningham, W., Fowler, M., . . . & Jeffries, R. (2001). *Manifesto for Agile software development*. The Agile Manifesto.

Berwick, D. M. (2003). Disseminating innovations in health care. *JAMA*, *289*(15), 1969–1975.

Bickmore, T. W., & Picard, R. W. (2005). Establishing and maintaining long-term human-computer relationships. *ACM Transactions on Computer-Human Interaction (TOCHI)*, *12*(2), 293–327.

Boehm, B. W. (1988). A spiral model of software development and enhancement. *Computer*, *21*(5), 61–72.

Botella, C., Gallego, M. J., Garcia-Palacios, A., Baños, R. M., Quero, S., & Alcañiz, M. (2009). The acceptability of an Internet-based self-help treatment for fear of public speaking. *British Journal of Guidance & Counselling*, *37*(3), 297–311.

Canzian, L., & Musolesi, M. (2015). Trajectories of depression: Unobtrusive monitoring of depressive states by means of smartphone mobility traces analysis. In *Proceedings of the 2015 ACM international joint conference on pervasive and ubiquitous computing*.

Cassell, J. (2001). Embodied conversational agents: Representation and intelligence in user interfaces. *AI Magazine*, *22*(4), 67.

Cassell, J., Bickmore, T., Campbell, L., Vilhjálmsson, H., & Yan, H. (2000). Conversation as a system framework: Designing embodied conversational agents. *Embodied Conversational Agents*, 29–63.

Chatterjee, S., & Price, A. (2009). Healthy living with persuasive technologies: Framework, issues, and challenges. *Journal of the American Medical Informatics Association*, *16*(2), 171–178.

De Montjoye, Y.-A., Hidalgo, C. A., Verleysen, M., & Blondel, V. D. (2013). Unique in the crowd: The privacy bounds of human mobility. *Scientific Reports*, *3*, 1376.

Diemer, J., Alpers, G. W., Peperkorn, H. M., Shiban, Y., & Mühlberger, A. (2015). The impact of perception and presence on emotional reactions: A review of research in virtual reality. *Frontiers in Psychology*, *6*.

Dingsøyr, T., Nerur, S., Balijepally, V., & Moe, N. B. (2012). A decade of agile methodologies: Towards explaining agile software development. *Journal of Systems and Software*, *85*(6), 1213–1221.

Eysenbach, G. (2001). What is e-health? *Journal of Medical Internet Research*, *3*(2), e20.

Ferrucci, D., Brown, E., Chu-Carroll, J., Fan, J., Gondek, D., Kalyanpur, A. A., . . . & Prager, J. (2010). Building Watson: An overview of the DeepQA project. *AI Magazine*, *31*(3), 59–79.

Fogg, B. J. (2002). Persuasive technology: Using computers to change what we think and do. *Ubiquity*, *2002*(December), 5.

Griffiths, F., Lindenmeyer, A., Powell, J., Lowe, P., & Thorogood, M. (2006). Why are health care interventions delivered over the internet? A systematic review of the published literature. *Journal of Medical Internet Research*, *8*(2), e10.

Hekler, E. B., Klasnja, P., Riley, W. T., Buman, M. P., Huberty, J., Rivera, D. E., & Martin, C. A. (2016). Agile science: Creating useful products for behavior change in the real world. *Translational Behavioral Medicine*, *6*(2), 317–328.

IJsselsteijn, W., de Kort, Y., Midden, C., Eggen, B., & van den Hoven, E. (2006). Persuasive technology for human well-being: Setting the scene. In W. A. Ijsselsteijn, Y. A. W. de Kort, C. Midden, B. Eggen, & E. van den Hoven (Eds.), *Proceedings of persuasive technology: First international conference on persuasive technology for human well-being, PERSUASIVE 2006, Eindhoven, The Netherlands, May 18–19, 2006* (pp. 1–5). Berlin, Heidelberg: Springer Berlin Heidelberg.

Kelders, S. M., Bohlmeijer, E. T., Pots, W. T., & van Gemert-Pijnen, J. E. (2015). Comparing human and automated support for depression: Fractional factorial randomized controlled trial. *Behaviour Research and Therapy*, *72*, 72–80.

Klein, J., Moon, Y., & Picard, R. W. (2002). This computer responds to user frustration: Theory, design, and results. *Interacting With Computers*, *14*(2), 119–140.

Ledger, D., & McCaffrey, D. (2014). Inside wearables: How the science of human behavior change offers the secret to long-term engagement. *Endeavour Partners*, *200*(93), 1.

Lee, J.-M., Kim, Y., & Welk, G. J. (2014). Validity of consumer-based physical activity monitors. *Medicine & Science in Sports & Exercise*, *46*(9), 1840–1848.

Lentferink, A. J., Oldenhuis, H. K. E., de Groot, M., Polstra, L., Velthuijsen, H., & van Gemert-Pijnen, J. E. W. C. (2017). Key components in eHealth interventions combining self-tracking and persuasive eCoaching to promote a healthier lifestyle: A scoping review. *Journal of Medical Internet Research*, *19*(8), e277.

Li, I., Dey, A. K., & Forlizzi, J. (2011). Understanding my data, myself: Supporting self-reflection with ubicomp technologies. In *Proceedings of the 13th international conference on ubiquitous computing*.

Munoz, A. (2014). *Machine learning and optimization*. Retrieved on March 2, 2016 from www.cims.nyu.edu/~munoz/files/ml_optimization.pdf [WebCite Cache ID 6fiLfZvnG].

Noar, S. M., Benac, C. N., & Harris, M. S. (2007). Does tailoring matter? Meta-analytic review of tailored print health behavior change interventions. *Psychological Bulletin*, *133*(4), 673.

North, M. M., & North, S. M. (2016). Virtual reality therapy. In *Computer-assisted and web-based innovations in psychology, special education, and health* (pp. 141–156). Amsterdam: Elsevier Inc.

Patel, M. S., Asch, D. A., & Volpp, K. G. (2015). Wearable devices as facilitators, not drivers, of health behavior change. *JAMA*, *313*(5), 459–460.

Patrick, K., Hekler, E. B., Estrin, D., Mohr, D. C., Riper, H., Crane, D., . . . & Riley, W. T. (2016). The pace of technologic change: implications for digital health behavior intervention research. *American Journal of Preventive Medicine*, *51*(5), 816–824.

Petersen, K., Wohlin, C., & Baca, D. (2009). The waterfall model in large-scale development. *Paper presented at the PROFES*.

Piwek, L., Ellis, D. A., Andrews, S., & Joinson, A. (2016). The rise of consumer health wearables: Promises and barriers. *PLoS Medicine*, *13*(2), e1001953.

Price, M., Mehta, N., Tone, E. B., & Anderson, P. L. (2011). Does engagement with exposure yield better outcomes? Components of presence as a predictor of treatment response for virtual reality exposure therapy for social phobia. *Journal of Anxiety Disorders*, *25*(6), 763–770.

Rothbaum, B. O., Hodges, L., Watson, B. A., Kessler, G. D., & Opdyke, D. (1996). Virtual reality exposure therapy in the treatment of fear of flying: A case report. *Behaviour Research and Therapy*, *34*(5), 477–481.

Scholten, M., Kelders, S. M., & van Gemert-Pijnen, J. E. W. C. (2017). Self-guided web-based interventions: A scoping review on user needs and on the potential of embodied conversational agents to address them. *Journal of Medical Internet Research*, *19*(11).

Schultheis, M. T., & Rizzo, A. A. (2001). The application of virtual reality technology in rehabilitation. *Rehabilitation Psychology*, *46*(3), 296.

Somashekhar, S. P., Kumarc, R., Rauthan, A., Arun, K. R., Patil, P., & Ramya, Y. E. (2017). *Abstract S6-07: Double blinded validation study to assess performance of IBM artificial intelligence platform, Watson for oncology in comparison with Manipal multidisciplinary tumour board – First study of 638 breast cancer cases: AACR*.

Swan, M. (2013). The quantified self: Fundamental disruption in big data science and biological discovery. *Big Data*, *1*(2), 85–99.

Talbot, F. (2012). Client contact in self-help therapy for anxiety and depression: Necessary but can take a variety of forms beside therapist contact. *Behaviour Change*, *29*(2), 63–76.

Tichon, J. G., & Mavin, T. (2016). Using the experience of evoked emotion in virtual reality to manage workplace stress: Affective Control Theory (ACT). In *Integrating technology in positive psychology practice* (pp. 344-362). Hershey, PA: IGI Global.
Turner, W. A., & Casey, L. M. (2014). Outcomes associated with virtual reality in psychological interventions: Where are we now? *Clinical Psychology Review, 34*(8), 634-644.

4

THE LIVED EXPERIENCE OF DIGITAL HEALTH

This chapter was first published in *Digital Health* and cross-referencing relates to chapters in the original volume. Please visit www.routledge.com/9781138123458 for more information about the book

The previous chapter outlined research investigating broad patterns in digital health technology use, with a particular focus on differences between social groups and geographical regions. The present chapter continues with examining digital health use, but moves into a different direction by discussing more in-depth research investigating people's lived experiences of digital health and implications for selfhood, embodiment and social relations. The discussion directs attention to how and why these technologies are used and actively incorporated into everyday life or otherwise resisted, rejected or ignored, and the sensory and emotional dimensions of these enactments and entanglements.

Social connection and emotion online

An important element of the ethos of contemporary online discussion forums and social media platforms is the expectation that users divulge details about themselves in collaborative efforts to establish social ties and a sense of community. The interactive affordances of online media, including the possibility of adopting an anonymous pseudonym on some platforms, promotes a culture of confession and sharing. Details about the self and the body that were once kept to the private sphere are now often broadcast online, often to potentially very large audiences (Banning 2016; John 2017). The affordances for social connections that online media offer are central to their emotional resonances and meanings.

A wealth of literature has demonstrated the value that patients have derived from being able to share their experiences on blogs and social media. The opportunity to engage with other people online can be immensely helpful and comforting. Many people go online because these technologies are so readily available and accessible any time of the day or night. People sometimes feel that they do not want to 'bother' healthcare providers with questions or concerns that may appear trivial, or find that access to face-to-face medical expertise is limited (Kraschnewski *et al.* 2014; Powell *et al.* 2011). As numerous studies have now shown, patients appreciate the greater access to information about their conditions and the reassurance, support, opportunity to express themselves, feeling part of a community and greater sense of control over their illness that they may gain from their participation in online forums and blogs (see, for example, Lee *et al.* 2014a; Mazanderani *et al.* 2013a, 2013b; McCosker and Darcy 2013; Powell *et al.* 2011; Ziebland and Wyke 2012). Online forums can also provide a place for people to express their grief at the serious illness or death of a loved one, thus providing them with an opportunity to talk about their feelings in ways that may be less socially accepted in face-to-face encounters (Chapple and Ziebland 2011; Gibson 2017).

Blogs and social media sites also help people who feel marginalised because of their health conditions, disability or their non-normative bodies to communicate with each other, find and give support and express their feelings. These media are used by people who identify as lesbian, bisexual, gay, transsexual or queer to find others to seek support or information, engage in activism or to develop friendships or sexual relationships (Fink and Miller 2014; O'Riordan and Phillips 2007; Pullen and Cooper 2010). Online forums and social media can be particularly helpful for people with illnesses that are stigmatised, such as HIV/AIDS or severe mental illness, providing opportunities to deal with feelings of social isolation and hopelessness (McDermott 2015; Mo and Coulson 2014; Naslund *et al.* 2014) or to discuss how medications affect them (Tucker and Goodings 2017).

My research with Sarah Pedersen on the ways in which pregnant women and mothers of young children used forums, social media and apps (Lupton 2016d; Lupton and Pedersen 2016; Pedersen and Lupton 2017) revealed that the women commonly went online to alleviate feelings of boredom, social isolation and distress. Immediate access to content was a priority for the majority of participants. The women referred to googling information constantly in an attempt to deal with worries or questions about pregnancy or their infants, and commented on the emotional relief they obtained when they could access advice from healthcare providers or other mothers online. They appreciated being able to connect to others at any time of the day or night. Our analysis of maternal feeling expressed on a popular parenting forum Mumsnet (Pedersen and Lupton 2017) showed that women expressed highly negative emotions about their experiences of motherhood. Contributors to the forum frequently noted that it was the only place they could express socially proscribed emotions such as anger, frustration, shame, guilt and sadness about motherhood and their children.

Social media affordances reinforce the emotional gratifications of interacting online. The ability to 'like', 'favourite', share, tag or comment on personal content provides an array of responses to other users. The practice of contributing to social media by posting updates or images or comments on other people's posts can be experienced as playful and pleasurable, as can observing the ways in which other users respond to one's posts and updates (Gerlitz and Helmond 2013; Grosser 2014). As observed in Chapter 4, the opportunity to engage as a 'good citizen' in sharing and pooling information that can benefit others is a major discourse on patient support platforms and online forums. Participants can gain satisfaction from contributing to scientific research, volunteering for clinical trials and the production of better understanding of their condition, as well as providing information and emotional support to other patients (Adams 2011; Harris *et al.* 2012; Mazanderani *et al.* 2013a; Tucker and Goodings 2017).

Not all people want to engage online, however. Studies of people living with cancer, for example, have discovered that some would rather avoid being confronted with a high level of detail about what may lie in store for them in terms of their treatment and prognosis, and therefore choose to avoid blogs, discussion groups and other online forums about cancer (Broom and Tovey 2008; Sandaunet 2008). People who are ill may also prefer not to represent this part of their lives to their social media friends and followers. Research involving interviews with Canadian teenagers hospitalised with chronic illness (Van Der Velden and El Emam 2013) identified that the participants were reluctant to reveal details of their illness on their Facebook accounts. These young people preferred to represent themselves as 'normal', healthy adolescents on Facebook, and used the platform as a way of escaping a focus on their illness. They were also reluctant to search for information about their conditions online or connect with other patients with their condition using digital media or with organisations related to their condition.

Another study interviewed people with diabetes and those attempting to lose weight and who were active users of online health forums and Facebook (Newman *et al.* 2011) The researchers found that, while participants were keen users of these platforms for support, advice, motivation and information-sharing purposes, they were confronted with constantly negotiating what type of details they should reveal. These participants were concerned about maintaining self-presentation in positive ways and were wary of boring other members with too much information about themselves. They thought carefully about what information about their health or weight loss they decided to share and with whom. These people wanted to present themselves as positive and helpful members of forums and also as actively managing their own health well. This meant that they did not necessarily want other members knowing about their struggles to engage in self-care (for diabetes) or their difficulties in achieving weight loss. Some topics, such as sexual health issues, may be considered simply too personal, sensitive or embarrassing to discuss on social media sites (Byron *et al.* 2013).

Nor do patients necessarily want access to all the medical information that their healthcare providers record about them. Interviews with British patients with a chronic illness (Winkelman *et al.* 2005) found that the information contained in the patients' electronic health records was limited in its usefulness. The patients observed that the doctors' accounts of their illness, as transcribed in the records, differed significantly from their own. This raises the question of clashing views of interpretation of their bodies from the patient compared with the health provider perspective and how these might be resolved. Some patients expressed the view that they did not necessarily want to be 'empowered' by being able to view all their information; they would rather not know about negative test findings or prognoses, for example, by reading it on the record before being able to discuss this information with their doctor.

It should also be acknowledged that a diversity of opinion is expressed by lay people who contribute to online health and medical sites. There may be disputes and disagreements with and outright hostility directed at other users. This is often the case, for example, on platforms or social media groups in which parents interact. Medical topics attracting strong opinions or emotions can provoke online arguments, as witnessed in discussions of childhood vaccination on a parenting forum (Skea *et al.* 2008). If participants hold different views from the majority of members of an online forum or Facebook health support group, they can find themselves shunned, castigated or asked to leave. Thus, for example, a study of a pro-anorexia online community found that participants were often challenged about their authenticity as 'pro-ana' advocates, labelled as 'wannarexics' or 'real' anorexics instead (Boero and Pascoe 2012).

People who are considered to lack the ability to engage in self-control and management of their health can be subjected to a high degree of moral opprobrium and abuse in online forums. This is a common experience of fat people (De Brún *et al.* 2014). It has also been encountered by people with cancer who openly admit that they smoke cigarettes (Luberto *et al.* 2016) and people with HIV/AIDS whose views differed from other members of online support groups (Mo and Coulson 2014). People from minority, marginalised or stigmatised social groups can find themselves discriminated against or simply not acknowledged on mainstream discussion forums and online support groups. As revealed in a study of Australian breast cancer information and support websites, women who were lesbian or from ethnic minority backgrounds were often not acknowledged or catered for (Gibson *et al.* 2016).

Online forums, therefore, work as important outlets for emotional expression and finding the support of likeminded others. However, they can also operate in highly normative ways, working to silence dissent and promote one set of opinions over others. Just as is the case with other avenues for the public discussion of health and illness matters, people who do not conform to accepted norms may find themselves marginalised. There is also the possibility that inaccurate, misleading or overly confronting information may be shared on these forums which may exacerbate rather than ameliorate health conditions and emotional wellbeing.

The emotional dimensions of digitised self-care

As in discourses attempting to represent the patient as a 'consumer' in earlier eras (Lupton 1997a, 1997b, 2012; Lupton *et al.* 1991), contemporary writings on patient engagement assume a rational, emotionally disengaged and 'empowered' subject who is motivated and equipped with the economic and cultural capital to engage in self-monitoring and self-care. In the discourse of the digitally engaged patient, 'empowerment' becomes a set of obligations (Veitch 2010). This perspective dominates in medical and popular representations of digitised patient self-care. Patients' resistance to the use of digital health devices for self-care is often explained by factors such as incompetence, indifference, ignorance or even technophobia (particularly in relation to older people). Yet even younger people, who are more experienced in the use of digital technologies more generally, may resent, challenge or simply ignore the tasks and responsibilities demanded of them by telemedicine. As Oudshoorn (2016: 767) has observed, while there are many 'heroic stories about the fusion of bodies and machines', very little literature on the entanglements of humans and medical technologies has paid attention to the vulnerabilities that such encounters may generate for people.

Taking on the ideals of the 'digitally engaged patient' is complex and can involve significant ambivalence for both patients and their healthcare professionals. Telemedical and telehealth devices have disciplinary and surveillant capabilities, making specific demands of patients and workers. Digital health technologies and the disciplinary regimes they configure as part of the practices of self-monitoring and self-care may be said both to empower and disempower patients. Researchers have commented on the 'invisible labour' required of patients in adapting self-care and other telecare technologies into their lives (Oudshoorn 2008, 2016; Piras and Miele 2017). Digital self-care technologies make specific demands of patients, requiring them to engage in self-monitoring practices at certain times of the day, for example, or beeping to remind them to take medication, or requesting them to rate and rank their healthcare providers on an evaluation website, or to upload their personal experiences of illness and medical treatment on patient support websites. Appropriating and incorporating any form of digital device into everyday life involves embodied practice and emotional responses. Users adopt ways of adjusting to wearing the devices, developing mundane embodied routines for attaching them, taking them off, ensuring that they are connected to the internet or other devices, responding to visual notifications and any haptic or auditory signals they send (such as buzzes or beeps) and ensuring that they are charged with power.

Medical technologies such as the insulin pump that are permanently implanted in bodies work to manage the body by monitoring it and also providing a substance that manages disease and maintains the user's health and bodily integrity. In a piece on 'hacking the feminist disabled body', Laura Forlano, a woman with diabetes who is also a feminist science and technologies studies academic, observes: 'At times, living with a chronic disease and disability such as diabetes can be a comedy of objects – a humorous negotiation between the human body and an entirely new set of actors [the apparatuses that are required to self-manage diabetes]' (Forlano 2016). Forlano acknowledges that her digital devices for managing diabetes are life-saving and health-giving. Having the insulin pump attached to her body provided her with reassurance and feelings of security and safety.

Kerry Sparling (2014), another woman with diabetes, wrote on her blog about how she has found that uploading her continuous blood glucose measurements to a cloud-based digital data archive meant that her husband and other family members could log in and check her data. The device is inserted under the user's skin on her stomach and the sensor within it constantly monitors blood glucose levels in body tissue fluid every few seconds and wirelessly transmits the data to a monitoring device worn or carried on the user's body. Sparling notes that if she were at home alone with her infant daughter or travelling, her family could check the data to ensure that she hadn't lapsed into a diabetic coma with no other adult present to help her.

As these women's accounts demonstrate, there are many possibilities for experiencing a sense of community and intimacy, reassurance and comfort from engaging with patient self-monitoring technologies. When patients think that they have achieved better knowledge of their bodies via self-monitoring devices they feel as if they are more in control and this leads to feelings of security and reassurance. However, if the data patients produce suggest that their health is suffering, or if these data conflict with their own subjective and phenomenological interpretation of their state of health and wellbeing, this can be unsettling and anxiety- or fear-provoking.

Many studies have demonstrated that the lived reality of tracking one's illness and engaging in self-care can simply be too confronting, tiring or depressing for people who are chronically or acutely ill. Self-monitoring and self-care for health and medical purposes become part of the burden of treatment with which patients are confronted. A Dutch study of people with diabetes (Hortensius *et al.* 2012) discovered that, while some of the interviewees described the self-monitoring technology they used as a 'friend', bestowing peace of mind, confidence, freedom and certainty, others represented it as a 'foe'. They disliked having to prick their finger constantly to elicit the blood for the test, and feeling ashamed, anxious, helpless or frustrated by glucose readings that were not in the appropriate range. Danish research (Huniche *et al.* 2013), investigating patients' experiences with self-monitoring their chronic obstructive pulmonary disease at home, found that the biometric readings these patients produced on their bodies, such as their oxygen saturation levels and lung function, were valued for their objectivity, their ability to uncover the mysteries of their bodies. The patients responded emotionally to the numerical data they produced, feeling encouraged, more secure or reassured when the numbers were in the acceptable range, but experiencing anxiety, depression or fear of physical deterioration when their data exceeded this range.

The dominant discourses idealising the engaged, self-responsible patient can lend a moralistic tenor to self-care practices. This was evident in an interview study with patients with multiple chronic conditions living in New York City (Ancker *et al.* 2015a, 2015b). Some patients did not wish to confront their biometric data, as it made them feel depressed, anxious, guilty or worried when 'bad numbers' appeared in their results. Spikes in blood glucose levels could happen for no apparent reason, and this was frustrating and demoralising for people who thought that they were managing their diabetes well. Personal biometric data were described by the patients in moralistic terms, as denoting that they had 'cheated' or somehow failed to maintain an appropriate health regimen if their data suggested this. Failing to engage consistently in self-tracking was also considered by the interviewees as evidence of being a 'bad patient' by failing to live up to healthcare providers' expectations of them, whereas those who were considered too thorough were also viewed negatively by healthcare providers, who described them as 'obsessive' or 'compulsive'. Some patients expressed their frustration or anger about being placed in a position where they had to focus on their disease continually, and would rather seek to forget that they were ill.

The pleasures and frustrations of self-tracking

For healthy people who are not dealing with illness or managing chronic conditions, self-tracking of elements of one's bodily functions and practices can be experienced as productive, empowering and playful. Via self-tracking initiatives, people are encouraged to generate information on themselves that can be used to optimise their lives and health status. Some self-trackers engage in competitive endeavours or see their self-tracking efforts as contributing to the aestheticisation and performance of parts of their lives. The opportunity to demonstrate to oneself, and perhaps also to others, that a self-tracker is becoming physically fitter, more productive, moving towards a weight-loss goal or beating a habit like smoking can be a powerful motivator. Many self-trackers who track their physical achievements and exploits using digital devices and then post their data to social media platforms or dedicated fitness tracking sites have identified their pleasure at being able to view and review the information about their activities, show them off to others and even compete against other users (Fotopoulou and O'Riordan 2017; Lupton 2016a: 201a, 2017b; Nafus and Sherman 2014; Ruckenstein 2014, 2015; Sharon and Zandbergen 2017; Smith and Vonthethoff 2017; Stragier *et al.* 2015; Sumartojo *et al.* 2016).

The acts of measuring and monitoring aspects of embodiment can significantly change the ways in which bodies are conceptualised and experienced, and also how people who engage in these activities are viewed by others. A wearable device such as a Fitbit can signal to others that the wearer is interested in his or her health and physical fitness as a symbolic object, whether or not the wearer is actually moving more or even pays any attention to the data the device generates. Alternatively, such a device or the presence of a fitness-monitoring app on a smartphone may be interpreted as evidence of obsessiveness, laziness or weakness, revealing the wearer's need to be disciplined and motivated by a technology rather than possessing internal willpower (Dennison *et al.* 2013) or that person's overenthusiastic interest in the numbers generated over other aspects of exercise (Copelton 2010).

For self-trackers, generating data about their body is an opportunity to acquire self-knowledge, engage in self-reflection and optimise their lives. Self-trackers often seek to make meaning from their data. The practice is not simply about collecting data but also attempting to engage with issues such as what should be done with these data, how they should be presented and interpreted and what the implications are for self-trackers' identity and future life prospects and success (Fotopoulou and O'Riordan 2017; Lupton 2017a; Lupton *et al.* 2017; Nafus and Sherman 2014; Smith and Vonthethoff 2017; Sumartojo *et al.* 2016). In so doing, self-trackers are engaging in voluntary self-surveillance. The process of meaning making may be facilitated by engaging in data-sharing practices. For those who participate in the communal mode of self-tracking (Lupton 2016a, 2017b), these data offer means of entering into exchanges of personal information for the mutual benefit of other users or the opportunity to contribute to aggregated big data sets that promise to reveal insights that may be of use to themselves and others (Barta and Neff 2016; Fotopoulou and O'Riordan 2017; Lomborg and Frandsen 2016; Lupton 2017b). When self-trackers engage in these practices, they are inviting the surveillance of others.

Mundane practices may be reconsidered as offering valuable contributions to accumulating metrics about heart rate or steps taken. Routine activities like strolling in the neighbourhood, walking or cycling to work or the shops or carrying out housework are reinterpreted as evidence of measurable bodily activity. Many people who use digital devices for monitoring their bodies find that the act of self-tracking and the data generated make them think about their bodies and their everyday physical activities differently.

A study of pedometer use in a USA-based walking group for adults aged over 50 is instructive (Copelton 2010). Pedometers are devices for measuring the number of steps taken. When this walking group was first formed, all participants were issued with a pedometer as a way of tracking their exercise patterns. However, resistance was identified among the members of the group to wearing the pedometers. It was contended by participants that these devices would interfere with sociability by introducing competitiveness and instituting a hierarchy of fitness into the group, and might place unwanted pressure on members to walk faster or longer. Wearing a pedometer upon one's body was viewed as an overt sign that one is monitoring oneself and thus placing emphasis on health or achievement over sociability. Hence these devices were quickly discarded.

A project involving young English men using smartphone apps to monitor their steps (Harries and Rettie 2016) came to similar conclusions concerning the ways in which monitoring walking using digital devices attracted new meanings. It was found that the participants' awareness that their physical activity was being tracked by the app resulted in them changing their habits. They tended to walk more in an attempt to increase their step metrics. Short walks that were part of their everyday movements received greater attention as opportunities to accumulate steps, transforming these walks into 'exercise'. Both this study and that undertaken by Copleton identified that moral meanings concerning responsible healthy citizenship and competitive and comparative impulses adhered to walking that was monitored and quantified, while non-tracked walking was invested with different meanings.

People often respond emotionally to their personal data when they view the visualisations that are produced from the data, such as graphs. A study of Finns using digital self-monitoring devices for physical activity and heart rate tracking (Pantzar and Ruckenstein 2015; Ruckenstein 2014) revealed that participants found the visualisations that were generated from their data meaningful and motivational, generating feelings of pride, accomplishment and satisfaction. The data visualisations were viewed as more credible and accurate by the participants than the 'subjective' assessments of their bodily sensations; indeed they expressed the desire for more data about their bodies to add to those already collected, so as to provide further insights.

My research investigating cycling self-tracking practices and meanings with Sarah Pink, Shanti Sumartojo and Christine Heyes Labond (Lupton *et al.* 2017; Sumartojo *et al.* 2016) discovered that people who monitored their cycling trips often invested emotionally in the data they generated. Quantified evidence that people were becoming fitter and faster when cycling proved to be highly motivating, lending confidence to people who had begun feeling unfit or incompetent at cycling. Several of the participants we talked to experienced much pleasure in reviewing their data and noting improvements in their speed or heart rate or noting that they had achieved 'personal bests' or trounced other users of the self-tracking platform they used for monitoring their rides. When data were lost due to a technical error or human forgetfulness (failing to charge up a device, for example) or if the details appeared inaccurate, people often reported feeling disappointed or frustrated.

As this study and others on self-tracking discussed here identify, digitised self-monitoring can have profound emotional resonances for those who take up these practices. Devoting time and attention to adopting a self-tracking practice and learning to make sense of the data it generates involves a continual assessment of how 'good' or 'valuable' these data are, what worth they have and how they should contribute to one's sense of self and embodiment. Like other self-care or self-monitoring practices, digitised self-tracking involves various forms of labour, including emotional, technical and sense-making work.

Spaces of digital health and surveillance

With the advent of mobile devices that can be carried or worn by users and insertible, implantable and ingestible sensors, not only has the clinic moved into the home, it has dispersed to every possible spatial and temporal location. Not only are medical and health-related data now mobile, but so are the bodies/devices that produce these data. As is the case with previous forms of telecare, many of the new digital health technologies are directed at repositioning healthcare, locating it within the domestic domain rather than the clinic and moving physical encounters of patients with healthcare providers to virtual encounters (Mort *et al.* 2009; Mort and Smith 2009; Oudshoorn 2011; 2012; Pols 2012). The home consequently becomes one node of a dispersed network of healthcare technologies in multiple sites and involving multiple actors who interpret the data supplied by telecare patients, diagnose and prescribe treatments and answer patients' queries.

With the use of digital health technologies like telemedicine and patient self-care devices, the 'medical gaze' is fragmented and distributed over different actors and locations (Nicolini 2007; Oudshoorn 2011, 2012; Pols 2012; Ruckenstein

2015). Medical care becomes simultaneously 'at a distance' (Oudshoorn 2008) and 'closer' than ever before by virtue of its surveillance capacities (Pols 2012). The spatial distance these technologies enact allows patients to avoid the direct medical gaze and disciplinary power that was the focus in Foucault's writings on the clinic (Chapter 1). However, this medical gaze becomes virtual and moves towards self-governance, as patients are expected to turn the gaze upon themselves and then report what they observe to their healthcare providers.

The techno-utopian ideals of the technologies used for these purposes are frequently challenged in the lived experiences of the patients who use them. As several sociologists of science and technology have discovered in their empirical work, while the assumed uses of telemedicine offer various defined possibilities, when they are actually put into use across a diverse range of contexts, the outcomes can be hard to predict. Merely providing the technologies to patients does not guarantee that they will be used as expected. Technologies like those used in patient self-care must be 'tamed' or 'tinkered with' to fit into patients' lives and operate usefully. They may end up being employed in ways that are very different from original expectations as users transform the technologies to make them meaningful (Nicolini 2007; Oudshoorn 2016; Pols 2012; Pols and Willems 2011).

People use various strategies to domesticate digital health technologies to render them more familiar and acceptable. In her analysis of the experiences of New Zealand patients using computerised self-dialysis technologies, Shaw (2015) used the term 'body-in-dialysis' to highlight the entanglements of digital machine and flesh that are configured when patients use their self-dialysis technologies at home. She observed that patients must carefully plan their daily and weekly routines around dialysis and ensure that a part of their homes is set up with all the equipment they need, including storage facilities for equipment such as boxes of fluid bags. Acknowledging a certain ambivalence about self-dialysis as both life-saving and overly dominating, patients personalised the dialysis machine, giving it human names and attributes such as personalities, describing the intimate, friendly relationships with their machines or alternatively noting the machine's tendency to 'misbehave' or act in controlling ways.

Some people find the obligation of self-surveillance in their homes to be frustrating and overwhelming. Thus, for example, research on Dutch heart patients using telemedicine devices such as a system to measure their body weight and blood pressure, a mobile phone capable of conducting and transmitting an electrocardiogram and a device to diagnose heart rhythm irregularities found that patients' bodies and home environments were disciplined by the routines expected of them. They were expected to conform to precise daily schedules of monitoring their bodies and sending data to their healthcare providers and to respond to messages and indicators sent to them at various times daily (Oudshoorn 2009, 2011, 2012). Oudshoorn (2011) discovered that some of the heart patients she studied who resisted using these technologies did so because they did not wish to have a constant reminder that they were ill and they resented the task of monitoring themselves constantly and having their homes transformed into a medical clinic. The surveillance offered by these technologies was thus positioned by these resistant users as restrictive of their autonomy, contributing to anxiety about their health or detracting from their preferred sense of selfhood and embodiment.

While some users experience self-monitoring or self-care technologies as restrictive and constraining of their autonomy, for others they afford the possibility to evade the medical gaze, to take control over their illness and their wayward body or to achieve independence. Some patients value these technologies as a way of avoiding a visit to the doctor when they would rather not see the doctor face to face, and thus establish a distance from medical surveillance (Andreassen *et al.* 2006). Patients may respond to the disciplinary and surveillance imperatives of self-care and self-monitoring by resisting or evading healthcare providers' directions and the obligations expected of them. Individuals may have other priorities and thus simply fail to use the devices provided them in the ways expected of them. Some patients 'play the system', experiment with their therapies or withdraw information from the healthcare providers if it does not conform to expectations (Nicolini 2007; Piras and Miele 2017).

However, there are limits to the extent to which people can resist or modify digital health technologies. Mol and Law (Mol 2009; Mol and Law 2004) conducted a study of Dutch people with diabetes who were required to monitor their blood glucose levels regularly throughout the day. They noted the complexities and difficulties of using self-monitoring technologies and in interpreting the data produced: 'in practice daily care turns around messy, material, smelly, bloody, frightening, or tedious activities that tend to be difficult to do (for professionals as well as patients)' (Mol 2009: 1756–1757). Mol points out that attempts to exercise control over the diabetic body, including the use of monitoring and self-care devices, are doomed to fail, simply because of the vagaries and erratic nature both of the body and the technologies designed to assist people to take control: '[t]echnology is never quite tamed. It doesn't offer control, and it changes along with the other elements of daily care practices' (Mol 2009: 1757).

Digital health technologies that are worn on or implanted in patients' bodies can continually announce their presence to the user, by rubbing against the skin, not fitting well and therefore feeling wrong, making disruptive noises or vibrating. Feminist technoscience critic Laura Forlano (2016) describes living with diabetes as involving continual decisions about what to eat, how to manage her insulin pump and continuous glucose monitor, how to dress in response to wearing the pump and the context of where she would be seen by others that day and how to respond to the readings that devices gave her about her body. She observes that the data flows that are generated by these devices are constantly disciplining as well as monitoring and therapeutically adjusting her body, provoking responses from her: 'As such, I am part of them, and they are part of me.'

Forlano (2016) recounts times when her sleep was disturbed by the continuous glucose monitor buzzing constantly during the night in response to a technical error. She contends that the constant adjustments, learning of technical knowledge and other responses required of her to manage her medical devices position her as a 'feminist hacker of my own cyborg body'. The perspective of the feminist hacker, she asserts, involves moving beyond techno-utopian discourses by drawing attention to the invisible labour, constant adjustments and responses and other embodied practices of using digital technologies.

As Forlano's narrative emphasises, people with chronic conditions like diabetes and kidney failure must engage in the constant invisible labour of negotiating and managing their devices and data. Sometimes these requirements can simply prove too demanding. The late health blogger and activist Jessie Gruman struggled with several chronic conditions as well as stomach cancer. She wrote in her blog (Gruman 2013) that she did not want to use apps that required time and effort to use, given that she was already facing a high load of self-care. Neither did she want to be 'nagged' by her smartphone or to collect detailed data that would simply be ignored by her doctor. In this blog piece, Gruman contended that:

> the things that apps do – remind us, nudge us, identify patterns for us, help us monitor symptoms, send data to our doctor for us – constitute tiny fragments of days that we spend gasping for breath in our chairs, lying on our couches in pain or forcing ourselves to slog through endless uncomfortable chores.

Digital health technologies potentially reconfigure the subject of surveillance and complicate the concept of the panoptic and medical gaze. Telemedicine disperses the spaces of medical care and also the medical gaze from well beyond the clinic into and beyond patients' homes. A patient self-care device worn on the body or positioned in a prominent place in the home can be a potent symbol of illness, marking out the user as unwell or unhealthy. The clinic and the normalising and assessing gaze of healthcare providers are incorporated into the everyday domestic spaces and practices of the lay person via these technologies.

The lack of personal contact in remote consultations or regimens of patient self-care can also present challenges to patients. I referred in the previous chapter to a survey conducted in seven countries which included asking people whether they preferred to use virtual consultations with doctors or face-to-face encounters. The survey found that, in each country, face-to-face encounters were preferred, as they were considered to offer higher-quality medical care (Accenture Consulting 2016a). Qualitative research has similarly shown that some people prefer to engage in physical rather than virtual encounters with healthcare providers, wanting what they view as a more personal interaction (Mort *et al.* 2009; Oudshoorn 2011).

Norwegian researchers (Andreassen 2011; Andreassen and Dyb 2010; Andreassen *et al.* 2006) found that patients may appreciate the opportunities that using telemedical technologies offer for communicating with healthcare professionals, particularly if they find it difficult to travel to seek face-to-face medical attention. However, trust remains an integral aspect of such use: without trust, communicating via technologies would not be effective. Indeed, trust may be even more important than in a face-to-face medical encounter, given the less personal nature of digital communication (Andreassen *et al.* 2006).

Several researchers have explored the use of digital health technologies by older people, including the use of monitoring digital devices such as motion detectors, tags or badges for people with dementia so that their movements might be kept track of without the need for physical restraints, sensors in beds and chairs which are able to monitor sleep patterns, weight and movement in individuals living in residential care, and 'smart floors' that can detect if a person has fallen. Some researchers have concluded that they may be regarded as enabling and empowering devices which are able to assist older people achieve better mobility, independence and feelings of security and allow them to achieve their goal of living at home longer (Brittain *et al.* 2010; Loe 2010; Long 2012). Others, however, warn against the possibilities of coercing older people to use these technologies and the detrimental possibilities of depriving them of face-to-face human contact if they are lonely and feeling isolated (Mort *et al.* 2013; Oudshoorn *et al.* 2016; Roberts *et al.* 2012).

Indeed, in a study on older people and telecare at home in the UK and Spain Mort and colleagues (2013) showed that their participants often expressed resentment about being required to use the technologies and even deliberately 'misused' them in order to provoke responses from caregivers or healthcare professionals that would involve a greater degree of human contact. Greenhalgh and colleagues (2013) talked to older British people with assisted living needs, and found that the digital technologies provided to them failed to meet their requirements. Their interviewees valued social relationships over technologies, and many felt socially isolated and lonely. At best, the digital devices that monitored their health and physical activity were viewed as useful sources of information; but they did not improve participants' wellbeing.

Some older people simply do not see a reason to use a particular digital health technology as it does not offer them any advantage or it clashes with their self-perceptions. Oudshoorn and colleagues (2016) conducted research on the design and development of a human interaction robot for use in caring for older people in their homes and Dutch older people's opinions about this idea. They point out that the prevailing discourse assumes homogeneity of this age group, with little recognition of their diversity (differences based on whether a person has a disability, health status, community links, gender, ethnicity and race, and so on). Oudshoorn and colleagues' findings demonstrate that the telecare technologies that have been designed for this group positioned them as 'a dependent and decrepit "other"' in need of and desiring assistance to achieve independence and self-responsibility for their health and wellbeing (Oudshoorn *et al.* 2016: 172). The Dutch people they spoke to were reluctant to position themselves in this way – or indeed, even to categorise themselves as 'old' – and therefore these robots held little attraction for them.

As these in-depth studies conducted in different sociocultural milieux demonstrate, the ways in which people take up – or challenge, resist or transform – digital health technologies take place as part of highly complex human–non-human assemblages. Designers, policy makers and healthcare providers may hold certain defined expectations about how these devices may be used, but these often do not recognise the shifting and heterogeneous lifeworlds which the devices enter. These devices have the potential to be lively – to be incorporated usefully into people's mundane practices and concepts of selfhood, embodiment and social relations and to allow them to enhance the capacities of their bodies and improve their health and wellbeing. However, if their affordances offer little of value to prospective users, or if such individuals fail to imagine how they can be incorporated into their lives or, indeed, view themselves as appropriate users, then this potential cannot be realised.

***

The research reviewed above has demonstrated the contingencies and compromises that are part of the use of digital health technologies by both patients and healthcare workers. Human actors respond to digital health technologies by shaping them to fit their domestic or work practices where they can. Technologies are thereby appropriated and domesticated as part of regular or everyday routines. However, humans may themselves be disciplined by the technologies at those points where the technologies are resistant to intervention or change. Furthermore, patients and lay people use digital health technologies in diverse and sometimes contradictory or ambivalent ways. It is not simply a matter of either taking up or rejecting these technologies: many people move between these two positions. Some technologies are embraced on some occasions, while others may be rejected or resisted. Their meanings and uses are not stable but rather are subject to change and contestation, depending on the context in which they are located and the other actors with which they interact. As I go on to demonstrate in the next chapter, these issues are also pertinent in the context of the work of healthcare professionals.

References

Accenture Consulting. (2016a) Accenture 2016 Consumer Survey on Patient Engagement. Accessed 13 July 2016. Available from www.accenture.com/t00010101T000000__w__/au-en/_acnmedia/Accenture/Conversion-Assets/DotCom/Documents/Local/au-en/PDF/1/Accenture-Patients-Want-A-Heavy-Dose-of-Digital-Research-Global-Report.pdf.

Adams, S. (2011) Sourcing the crowd for health services improvement: the reflexive patient and 'share-your-experience' websites. Social Science & Medicine, 72 (7), 1069–1076.

Ancker, J., Witteman, H., Hafeez, B., Provencher, T., Van de Graaf, M. and Wei, E. (2015a) "You get reminded you're a sick person": personal data tracking and patients with multiple chronic conditions. Journal of Medical Internet Research (8). Accessed 30 August 2015. Available from www.jmir.org/2015/8/e202/?trendmd-shared=0.

Ancker, J., Witteman, H., Hafeez, B., Provencher, T., Van de Graaf, M. and Wei, E. (2015b) The invisible work of personal health information management among people with multiple chronic conditions: qualitative interview study among patients and providers. Journal of Medical Internet Research (6). Accessed 30 August 2015. Available from www.jmir.org/2015/6/e137/?trendmd-shared=0.

Andreassen, H. (2011) What does an e-mail address add? Doing health and technology at home. Social Science & Medicine, 72 (4), 521–528.

Andreassen, H. and Dyb, K. (2010) Differences and inequalities in health: empirical reflections on telemedicine and politics. Information, Communication & Society, 13 (7), 956–975.

Andreassen, H., Trondsen, M., Kummervold, P.E., Gammon, D. and Hjortdahl, P. (2006) Patients who use e-mediated communication with their doctor: new constructions of trust in the patient–doctor relationship. Qualitative Health Research, 16 (2), 238–248.

Banning, M.E. (2016) Shared entanglements – Web 2.0, info-liberalism & digital sharing. Information, Communication & Society, 19 (4), 489–503.

Barta, K. and Neff, G. (2016) Technologies for sharing: lessons from Quantified Self about the political economy of platforms. Information, Communication & Society, 19 (4), 518–531.

Boero, N. and Pascoe, C.J. (2012) Pro-anorexia communities and online interaction: bringing the pro-ana body online. Body & Society, 18 (2), 27–57.

Brittain, K., Corner, L., Robinson, L. and Bond, J. (2010) Ageing in place and technologies of place: the lived experience of people with dementia in changing social, physical and technological environments. Sociology of Health & Illness, 32 (2), 272–287.

Broom, A. and Tovey, P. (2008) The role of the internet in cancer patients' engagement with complementary and alternative treatments. Health:, 12 (2), 139–155.

Byron, P., Albury, K. and Evers, C. (2013) "It would be weird to have that on Facebook": young people's use of social media and the risk of sharing sexual health information. Reproductive Health Matters, 21 (41), 35–44.

Chapple, A. and Ziebland, S. (2011) How the internet is changing the experience of bereavement by suicide: a qualitative study in the UK. Health:, 15 (2), 173–187.

Copelton, D. (2010) Output that counts: pedometers, sociability and the contested terrain of older adult fitness walking. Sociology of Health & Illness, 32 (2), 304–318.

De Brún, A., McCarthy, M., McKenzie, K. and McGloin, A. (2014) Weight stigma and narrative resistance evident in online discussions of obesity. Appetite, 72, 73–81.

Dennison, L., Morrison, L., Conway, G. and Yardley, L. (2013) Opportunities and challenges for smartphone applications in supporting health behavior change: qualitative study. Journal of Medical Internet Research (4). Accessed 8 April 2014. Available from www.jmir.org/2013/4/e86/.

Fink, M. and Miller, Q. (2014) Trans media moments: Tumblr, 2011–2013. Television & New Media, 15 (7), 611–626.

Forlano, L. (2016) Hacking the feminist disabled body. Journal of Peer Production (8). Accessed 28 April 2016. Available from http://peerproduction.net/issues/issue-8-feminism-and-unhacking/peer-reviewed-papers/hacking-the-feminist-disabled-body/.

Fotopoulou, A. and O'Riordan, K. (2017) Training to self-care: fitness tracking, biopedagogy and the healthy consumer. Health Sociology Review, 26 (1), 54–68.

Gerlitz, C. and Helmond, A. (2013) The like economy: social buttons and the data-intensive web. New Media & Society, 15 (8), 1348–1365.

Gibson, A., Lee, C. and Crabb, S. (2016) Representations of women on Australian breast cancer websites: cultural 'inclusivity' and marginalisation. Journal of Sociology, 52 (2), 433–452.

Gibson, M. (2017) YouTube and bereavement vlogging: emotional exchange between strangers. Journal of Sociology, 52 (4), 631–645.

Greenhalgh, T., Wherton, J., Sugarhood, P., Hinder, S., Procter, R. and Stones, R. (2013) What matters to older people with assisted living needs? A phenomenological analysis of the use and non-use of telehealth and telecare. Social Science & Medicine, 93, 86–94.

Grosser, B. (2014) What do metrics want? How quantification prescribes social interaction on Facebook. Computational Culture. Accessed 16 November 2014. Available from http://computationalculture.net/article/what-do-metrics-want.

Gruman, J. (2013) What patients want from mobile apps. Accessed 9 April 2013. Available from www.kevinmd.com/blog/2013/04/patients-mobile-apps.html.

Harries, T. and Rettie, R. (2016) Walking as a social practice: dispersed walking and the organisation of everyday practices. Sociology of Health & Illness, 38 (6), 874–883.

Harris, A., Wyatt, S. and Kelly, S.E. (2012) The gift of spit (and the obligation to return it). Information, Communication & Society, 16 (2), 236–257.

Hortensius, J., Kars, M., Wierenga, W., Kleefstra, N., Bilo, H. and van der Bijl, J. (2012) Perspectives of patients with type 1 or insulin-treated type 2 diabetes on self-monitoring of blood glucose: a qualitative study. BMC Public Health (1). Accessed 5 May 2013. Available from www.biomedcentral.com/1471–2458/12/167.

Huniche, L., Dinesen, B., Nielsen, C., Grann, O. and Toft, E. (2013) Patients' use of self-monitored readings for managing everyday life with COPD: a qualitative study. Telemedicine and e-Health, 19 (5), 396–402.

John, N. (2017) The Age of Sharing. Cambridge: Polity.

Kraschnewski, L.J., Chuang, H.C., Poole, S.E., Peyton, T., Blubaugh, I., Pauli, J., Feher, A. and Reddy, M. (2014) Paging "Dr. Google": does technology fill the gap created by the prenatal care visit structure? Qualitative focus group study with pregnant women. Journal of Medical Internet Research (6). Accessed 17 July 2014. Available from www.jmir.org/2014/6/e147/.

Lee, K., Hoti, K., Hughes, D.J. and Emmerton, L. (2014a) Dr Google and the consumer: a qualitative study exploring the navigational needs and online health information-seeking behaviors of consumers with chronic health conditions. Journal of Medical Internet Research (12). Accessed 25 May 2016. Available from www.jmir.org/2014/12/e262/.

Loe, M. (2010) Doing it my way: old women, technology and wellbeing. Sociology of Health & Illness, 32 (2), 319–334.

Lomborg, S. and Frandsen, K. (2016) Self-tracking as communication. Information, Communication & Society, 19 (7), 1015–1017.

Long, S.O. (2012) Bodies, technologies, and aging in Japan: thinking about old people and their silver products. Journal of Cross-Cultural Gerontology, 27 (2), 119–137.

Luberto, C.M., Hyland, K.A., Streck, J.M., Temel, B. and Park, E.R. (2016) Stigmatic and sympathetic attitudes toward cancer patients who smoke: a qualitative analysis of an online discussion board forum. Nicotine & Tobacco Research, 18 (12), 2194–2201.

Lupton, D. (1997a) Consumerism, reflexivity and the medical encounter. Social Science & Medicine, 45 (3), 373–381.

Lupton, D. (1997b) Foucault and the medicalisation critique. In A. Petersen and R. Bunton (eds) Foucault, Health and Medicine. London: Routledge, 94–110.

Lupton, D. (2012) Medicine as Culture: Illness, Disease and the Body. 3rd ed. London: Sage.

Lupton, D. (2016a) The Quantified Self: A Sociology of Self-Tracking. Cambridge: Polity Press.

Lupton, D. (2016d) The use and value of digital media information for pregnancy and early motherhood: a focus group study. BMC Pregnancy and Childbirth, 16 (171). Accessed 5 December 2016. Available from http://bmcpregnancychildbirth.biomedcentral.com/articles/10.1186/s12884-016-0971-3.

Lupton, D. (2017a) Personal data practices in the age of lively data. In J. Daniels, K. Gregory and T. McMillan Cottom (eds) Digital Sociologies. Bristol: Policy Press, 339–354.

Lupton, D. (2017b) Lively data, social fitness and biovalue: the intersections of health self-tracking and social media. In J. Burgess, A. Marwick and T. Poell (eds) The Sage Handbook on Social Media. London: Sage, in press.

Lupton, D., Donaldson, C. and Lloyd, P. (1991) Caveat emptor or blissful ignorance? Patients and the consumerist ethos. Social Science & Medicine, 33 (5), 559–568.

Lupton, D. and Pedersen, S. (2016) An Australian survey of women's use of pregnancy and parenting apps. Women and Birth, 29 (4), 368–375.

Lupton, D., Pink, S., Labond, C.H. and Sumartojo, S. (2017) Personal data contexts, data sense and self-tracking cycling. International Journal of Communication, in press.

Mazanderani, F., Locock, L. and Powell, J. (2013a) Biographical value: towards a conceptualisation of the commodification of illness narratives in contemporary healthcare. Sociology of Health & Illness, 35 (6), 891–905.

Mazanderani, F., O'Neill, B. and Powell, J. (2013b) 'People power' or 'pester power'? YouTube as a forum for the generation of evidence and patient advocacy. Patient Education and Counseling, 93 (3), 420.

McCosker, A. and Darcy, R. (2013) Living with cancer: affective labour, self-expression and the utility of blogs. Information, Communication & Society, 16 (8), 1266–1285.

McDermott, E. (2015) Asking for help online: lesbian, gay, bisexual and trans youth, self-harm and articulating the 'failed' self. Health:. 19 (6), 561–577.

Mo, P.K.H. and Coulson, N.S. (2014) Are online support groups always beneficial? A qualitative exploration of the empowering and disempowering processes of participation within HIV/AIDS-related online support groups. International Journal of Nursing Studies, 51 (7), 983–993.

Mol, A. (2009) Living with diabetes: care beyond choice and control. Lancet, 373 (9677), 1756–1757.

Mol, A. and Law, J. (2004) Embodied action, enacted bodies: the example of hypoglycaemia. Body & Society, 10 (2–3), 43–62.

Mort, M., Finch, T. and May, C. (2009) Making and unmaking telepatients: identity and governance in new health technologies. Science, Technology & Human Values, 34 (1), 9–33.

Mort, M., Roberts, C. and Callén, B. (2013) Ageing with telecare: care or coercion in austerity? Sociology of Health & Illness, 35 (6), 799–812.

Mort, M. and Smith, A. (2009) Beyond information: intimate relations in sociotechnical practice. Sociology, 43 (2), 215–231.

Nafus, D. and Sherman, J. (2014) This one does not go up to 11: the Quantified Self movement as an alternative big data practice. International Journal of Communication, 8, 1785–1794.

Naslund, J.A., Grande, S.W., Aschbrenner, K.A. and Elwyn, G. (2014) Naturally occurring peer support through social media: the experiences of individuals with severe mental illness using YouTube. PloS One (10). Accessed 24 April 2016. Available from http://journals.plos.org/plosone/article?id=10.1371/journal.pone.0110171.

Newman, M.W., Lauterbach, D., Munson, S.A., Resnick, P. and Morris, M.E. (2011) It's not that I don't have problems, I'm just not putting them on Facebook: challenges and opportunities in using online social networks for health. *Proceedings of the ACM 2011 Conference on Computer Supported Cooperative Work* (CSCS '11). Hangzou: ACM Press, 341–350.

Nicolini, D. (2007) Stretching out and expanding work practices in time and space: the case of telemedicine. Human Relations, 60 (6), 889–920.

O'Riordan, K. and Phillips, D.J., eds. (2007) Queer Online: Media Technology & Sexuality. New York: Peter Lang.

Oudshoorn, N. (2008) Diagnosis at a distance: the invisible work of patients and healthcare professionals in cardiac telemonitoring technology. Sociology of Health & Illness, 30 (2), 272–288.

Oudshoorn, N. (2009) Physical and digital proximity: emerging ways of health care in face-to-face and telemonitoring of heart-failure patients. Sociology of Health & Illness, 31 (3), 390.

Oudshoorn, N. (2011) Telecare Technologies and the Transformation of Healthcare. Houndmills: Palgrave Macmillan.

Oudshoorn, N. (2012) How places matter: telecare technologies and the changing spatial dimensions of healthcare. Social Studies of Science, 42 (1), 121–142.

Oudshoorn, N. (2016) The vulnerability of cyborgs: the case of ICD shocks. Science, Technology & Human Values, 41(5), 767–792.

Oudshoorn, N., Neven, L. and Stienstra, M. (2016) How diversity gets lost: age and gender in design practices of information and communication technologies. Journal of Women & Aging, 28 (2), 170–185.

Pantzar, M. and Ruckenstein, M. (2015) The heart of everyday analytics: emotional, material and practical extensions in self-tracking market. Consumption Markets & Culture, 18 (1), 92–109.

Pedersen, S. and Lupton, D. (2017) 'What are you feeling right now?' Communities of maternal feeling on Mumsnet. Emotion, Space and Society, online ahead of print.
Piras, E.M. and Miele, F. (2017) Clinical self-tracking and monitoring technologies: negotiations in the ICT-mediated patient–provider relationship. Health Sociology Review, 26 (1), 38–53.
Pols, J. (2012) Care at a Distance: On the Closeness of Technology. Amsterdam: Amsterdam University Press.
Pols, J. and Willems, D. (2011) Innovation and evaluation: taming and unleashing telecare technology. Sociology of Health & Illness, 33 (3), 484–498.
Powell, J., Inglis, N., Ronnie, J. and Large, S. (2011) The characteristics and motivations of online health information seekers: cross-sectional survey and qualitative interview study. Journal of Medical Internet Research (1). Accessed 25 March 2016. Available from www.jmir.org/2011/1/e20/.
Pullen, C. and Cooper, M., eds. (2010) LGBT Identity and Online New Media. New York: Routledge.
Roberts, C., Mort, M. and Milligan, C. (2012) Calling for care: 'disembodied' work, teleoperators and older people living at home. Sociology, 46 (3), 490–506.
Ruckenstein, M. (2014) Visualized and interacted life: personal analytics and engagements with data doubles. Societies, 4 (1), 68–84.
Ruckenstein, M. (2015) Uncovering everyday rhythms and patterns: food tracking and new forms of visibility and temporality in health care. In L. Botin, C. Nohr and P. Bertelsen (eds) Techno-Anthropology in Health Informatics. Amsterdam: IOS Press, 28–40.
Sandaunet, A.G. (2008) The challenge of fitting in: non-participation and withdrawal from an online self-help group for breast cancer patients. Sociology of Health & Illness, 30 (1), 131–144.
Sharon, T. and Zandbergen, D. (2017) From data fetishism to quantifying selves: self-tracking practices and the other values of data. New Media & Society, online ahead of print.
Shaw, R. (2015) Being-in-dialysis: the experience of the machine–body for home dialysis users. Health:, 19 (3), 229–244.
Skea, Z.C., Entwistle, V.A., Watt, I. and Russell, E. (2008) 'Avoiding harm to others' considerations in relation to parental measles, mumps and rubella (MMR) vaccination discussions – an analysis of an online chat forum. Social Science & Medicine, 67 (9), 1382–1390.
Smith, G.J.D. and Vonthethoff, B. (2017) Health by numbers? Exploring the practice and experience of datafied health. Health Sociology Review, 26 (1), 6–21.
Sparling, K. (2014) CGM in the cloud: personal preferences. *Six Until Me*. Accessed 8 July 2016. Available from http://sixuntilme.com/wp/2014/07/16/cgm-cloud-personal-preferences.
Stragier, J., Evens, T. and Mechant, P. (2015) Broadcast yourself: an exploratory study of sharing physical activity on social networking sites. Media International Australia, 155 (1), 120–129.
Sumartojo, S., Pink, S., Lupton, D. and LaBond, C.H. (2016) The affective intensities of datafied space. Emotion, Space and Society, 21, 33–40.
Tucker, I. and Goodings, L. (2017) Medicated bodies: mental distress, social media and affect. New Media & Society, online ahead of print.
Van Der Velden, M. and El Emam, K. (2013) "Not all my friends need to know": a qualitative study of teenage patients, privacy, and social media. Journal of the American Medical Informatics Association, 20 (1), 16–21.
Veitch, K. (2010) The government of health care and the politics of patient empowerment: New Labour and the NHS reform agenda in England. Law & Policy, 32 (3), 313–331.
Winkelman, W.J., Leonard, K.J. and Rossos, P.G. (2005) Patient-perceived usefulness of online electronic medical records: employing grounded theory in the development of information and communication technologies for use by patients living with chronic illness. Journal of the American Medical Informatics Association, 12 (3), 306–314.
Ziebland, S. and Wyke, S. (2012) Health and illness in a connected world: how might sharing experiences on the internet affect people's health? Milbank Quarterly, 90 (2), 219–249.

CHAPTER 5
ENVIRONMENT- AND POLICY-BASED APPROACHES TO HEALTH BEHAVIOR CHANGE

This chapter was first published in *Health Behavior Change* and cross-referencing relates to chapters in the original volume. Please visit www.routledge.com/9781138694828 for more information about the book

OVERVIEW

In this chapter we examine the role of environmental factors and policies that influence health behaviors. Various aspects of the environment might be expected to influence our behavior. For example, a lack of suitable exercise facilities in the local area can impact on even the most fervent exerciser. Similarly, a lack of financial resources can prevent individuals from buying healthier but more expensive foods and consumer products. However, these influences of the environment can have effects on behavior either directly (where a mediating variable is not proposed, is automatic/unconscious, or there is no evidence of a mediating variable), indirectly (mediated effects) or by interacting with cognitions (moderation effects). In this chapter we consider these direct, mediated and moderated effects by which environmental factors may influence our behavior. Under direct paths we explore and examine nudge theory and choice architecture as a research area that has examined how making changes to our environment (broadly defined) might change our behavior. Under mediated paths we look at research on how changes in the environment may produce changes in cognitions, such as social norms or intentions, which in turn produce changes in behavior. Under moderated paths we look at how aspects of the environment may interact with cognitions to produce behavior. We then consider the effects of public policy-based solutions and social marketing approaches in changing behavior.

USING CLASSIC AND SOCIAL/HEALTH COGNITION MODELS

The behaviorist approach considered in Chapter 2 has always focused on external, environmental reinforcement contingencies as primary explanations for behavior and behavior change. The simple formula is: change the reinforcement schedule or behavioral cost, and you will see a change in the behavior. This approach is direct in nature and is similar to nudging behavior (which we overview later in this chapter) which impacts behavior via non-conscious processes, because deliberative or reflective cognitive processes need not be invoked or involved in changing behavior. By changing the accessibility, availability, desirability or cost of performing certain behavioral alternatives, corresponding changes in the behaviors should be observed.

In support of this behavioral approach, Faith, Rose, Matz, Pietrobelli and Epstein (2006) randomly assigned sets of 5-year-old twins to a treatment or control condition, one twin in each condition. In the contingent rewards condition, children were told that, for each serving of fruits or vegetables that they selected in their lunch, they would receive a voucher that could be exchanged for prizes at a later time. In the non-contingent rewards (control) condition, the children were told that they would receive a set of vouchers for prizes during lunch, but were not told that they were based on selecting certain types of food. Compared to their baseline eating behavior, twins in the contingent rewards group significantly increased their consumption of vegetables and fruits, and decreased their consumption of total energy and fat. Children in the control condition did not change their eating behavior compared to baseline levels. Findings such as these illustrate the power of positive reinforcement as an environmental variable that can increase healthier eating behaviors and other positive health behaviors.

The environment has also played a prominent role in some social/health cognition models, albeit in different ways. For instance, in the major theorist model (Fishbein et al., 2001; see Chapter 2), the environment is assumed to have a **direct effect** on behavior, facilitating behavior or preventing action even when the individual has the necessary skills and intentions. In contrast, in the Social Cognitive Theory (see Chapter 2), environmental factors are assumed to only influence behavior indirectly through changing goals or intentions, which in turn influence behavior (i.e., an **indirect/ mediated effect**).

Many social/health cognition models have been used to inform environment-based interventions. For example, in the area of social marketing (discussed in detail later in this chapter), Luca and Suggs (2013) reported that the most common theories used to develop social marketing interventions were the Stages of Change/Transtheoretical model (e.g., Prochaska & DiClemente, 1986; see also Gallivan, Lising, Ammary & Greenberg, 2007; Richert, Webb, Morse, O'Toole & Brownson, 2007) and the Theory of Reasoned Action/Theory of Planned Behavior (e.g., Ajzen, 1991; Fishbein & Ajzen, 1975; see also Long, Taubenheim, Wayman, Temple & Ruoff, 2008; Peterson, Abraham & Waterfield, 2005). However, they report that the majority of interventions in their review were not clearly designed according to any theoretical framework. Several studies did discuss theoretical models or frameworks, but did not discuss clearly or at all *how* the theory was used in designing their intervention. As we discussed in Chapter 4, this has important implications for how the results can and should be interpreted and used in future research.

DIRECT ENVIRONMENTAL IMPACTS ON BEHAVIOR

NUDGE THEORY AND CHOICE ARCHITECTURE

Thaler and Sunstein (2008) are behavioral economists whose book *Nudge: Improving Decisions about Health, Wealth, and Happiness* has been influential in attempts to change behavior based on changing aspects of the environment. They focus on the impact of the environment on decisions and behaviors. They suggest that we do not make choices in a vacuum but in an environment where many features of that environment influence our decisions. It is assumed that many of these environmental features are designed to influence behavior directly, outside of conscious awareness. Others are more transparent and require more cognitive and behavioral effort to have their effect.

Thaler and Sunstein use the term **choice architecture** to describe the creation or modification of aspects of the environment that influence choices. *Nudge* attempts to show how choice architecture can be used to help influence people into making certain choices using a variety of tools. The authors have created a website (www.nudges.org) where they describe various strategies under headings such as defaults, expecting error, giving feedback and creating incentives. For example, the idea of changing defaults from an 'opt in' default to an 'opt out' default has been shown to be successful in changing different types of behavior for quite some time now. One famous example by Johnson and Goldstein (2003) shows that by making organ donation consent the default option (compared to the requirement that potential donors exert the effort to opt in to the donation program), donation rates increase dramatically. To cite some specific cases, *opt-out* countries such as Sweden and Austria reported significantly higher numbers of donors (85.9% and 99.98%, respectively), compared to *opt-in* countries such as Denmark, the Netherlands and the UK (4.25%, 27.5% and 17.17%, respectively).

Since the publication of *Nudge* and related work, there have been several attempts to test the ideas scientifically in socially important contexts. For example, a team of researchers (see Levy, Riis, Sonnenberg, Barraclough & Thorndike, 2012; Thorndike, Sonnenberg, Riis, Barraclough & Levy, 2012; Thorndike, Riis, Sonnenberg & Levy, 2014) tested some relevant nudges and choice architecture interventions to decrease the likelihood of employees purchasing high-calorie foods and to increase the likelihood of their purchasing healthier foods. In one of their studies, they created a nine-month longitudinal design with interventions introduced sequentially. First, after a baseline period, they introduced food labels with a traffic light signal theme. Foods were labeled as 'green' (healthy), 'yellow/amber' (neutral) or 'red' (unhealthy/high calorie). Three months after the traffic light scheme had been introduced, they then used choice architecture to make 'green' choices more available and accessible, and to make the 'red' choices less available and accessible. Following their interventions they found significant reductions in 'red' choices, especially for 'red' (high calorie) beverages, which were reduced by 39%. In addition, most of their changes were sustained over two years post-intervention. In another study, Hanks, Just, Smith and Wansink, (2012) tested the idea of a 'convenience line' in addition to standard cafeteria lines in a school. In the convenience line students could only purchase healthy items (e.g., salads, sandwiches, fruits, and vegetables). This additional convenience line resulted in a significant reduction in the purchase of unhealthy foods. These studies illustrate the power of choice architecture in influencing healthier eating behaviors.

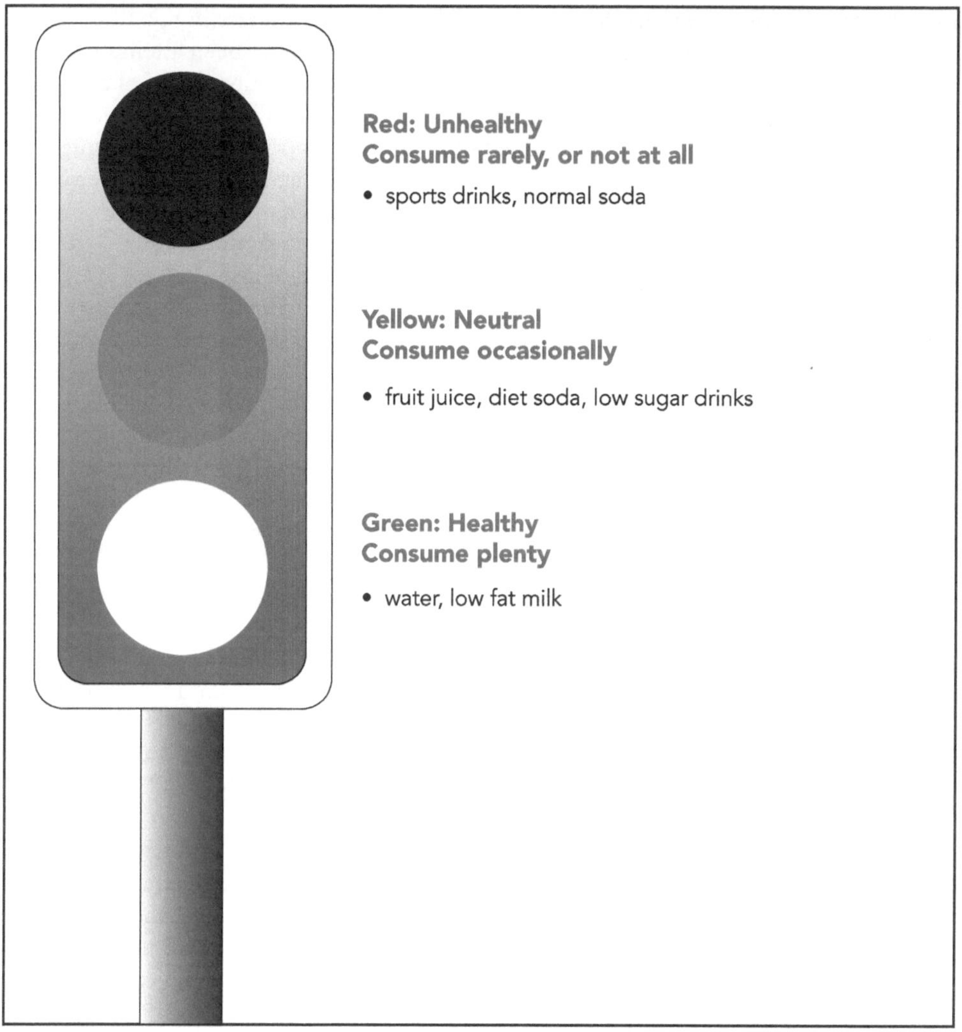

FIGURE 9.1 Images such as this one are used to nudge people in the direction of healthy food choices
Note: Red shown as black, yellow shown as gray and green shown as white.

A related intervention was undertaken in a Florida public school lunch program (see Miller, Gupta, Kropp, Grogan & Mathews, 2016). In this study, two interventions were compared to a control condition. The first intervention required that students use an online pre-ordering system for their lunches, whereas the second intervention used the same pre-ordering system along with behavioral nudges, which helped students to order a balanced and healthy meal. Specifically, students were prompted to order one element of each from among fruits, vegetables, whole grains, dairy and a main entrée. The second intervention yielded the best outcomes overall, compared to both other conditions. Specifically, students using the program with behavioral nudges for ordering more balanced meals did in fact select more fruits, vegetables and low fat milk with their lunches.

A variety of other interventions that target small but effective changes in the environment as a means to nudge or change behavior directly have been attempted. For example, Grant and Hofmann (2011) used a very simple manipulation of a sign about hand hygiene to change behavior among health professionals in a hospital. In study 1, one of three messages was randomly assigned to be displayed next to hand-sanitizing gel dispensers around the hospital. The control sign read, 'Gel in, wash out'; the personal consequences sign read, 'Hand hygiene prevents you from catching diseases'; the patient-consequences sign read, 'Hand hygiene prevents patients from catching diseases.' Based on measuring the amount of gel used, the rates of dispenser use were 40.1%, 34.0% and 54.2% respectively for the three groups showing that the message emphasizing patient consequences and presumably cueing professional behavior was most effective. In a second study, the personal consequences and patient consequences signs were compared using covert, independent observation. The rates of hand-hygiene adherence in the two groups were almost identical at baseline but 9.5% higher in the patient compared to personal consequences condition (89.2% vs. 79.7% adherence) at follow-up. These findings are a striking demonstration of how a simple manipulation (in this case changing one word) can produce significant changes in behavior.

How do people feel about nudges?

As we noted above, some of the environmental cues or nudges that influence behavior are largely outside of our awareness, whereas others are more visible and require more conscious, deliberate decision-making. Some researchers (e.g., Jung & Mellers, 2016; Kahneman, 2011) have used the terms **System 1 thinking** and **System 2 thinking** to refer to these types of nudges, respectively (see also Strack & Deutsch, 2004, for a discussion of a similar model, called the Reflective-Impulsive Model also covered in Chapters 2 and 8). That is, System 1 nudges tend to have more of an automatic or impulsive influence on behavior. Examples of this type of nudge include automatic enrollment into an organ donation program, smaller portions of food and changes in the visibility and accessibility of food items in shops or cafeterias. System 2 nudges, by comparison, require more effort, deliberation and reflection. For example, System 2 nudges might include food labels, nutritional information charts and overt prompts to make different food selections. These types of nudges can provide education and information enabling individuals to make more informed choices. So, when consumers are made aware of these different types of nudges influencing their behavior, how do they feel about them? One hypothesis is that people may feel that nudges are an attempt to control or manipulate their behavior, reacting negatively and resisting the nudge attempt, especially if those nudges are of the System 1 type.

In a US sample of adults, Jung and Mellers (2016) explored the role of individual differences in support for different types of nudges, and found some interesting patterns. First, there was general support for nudges to increase the likelihood of positive behaviors, but stronger support was obtained for System 2 (informational) nudges than for System 1 (automatic/default) nudges. Concerning individual differences, or preferences based on dispositional variables, empathetic people showed support for both types of nudges, especially when they were framed as have societal benefits. People scoring high on individualism and politically conservative respondents were unfavorable towards both types of nudges. Participants with high scores on a scale of reactance (e.g., 'I become frustrated when I am unable to make free and independent decisions' and 'When someone forces me to do something, I feel like doing the opposite'; see Hong & Page, 1989) and who reported a strong desire for control were primarily against System 1 nudges, and mediation models showed that the key determining factors in their resistance to such nudges were feelings that their autonomy was threatened by such nudges, and that such nudges were too paternalistic.

In samples of adults in both the UK and the US, Petrescu, Hollands, Couturier, Ng and Marteau (2016) asked respondents about the acceptability of a variety of interventions, based on nudging or choice architecture, to reduce obesity. These interventions, such as reducing portion sizes, changing the size and shape of containers, and making foods differentially accessible to consumers, included both System 1 and System 2 type nudges. In both the UK and US samples, respondents showed a preference for educational interventions (System 2 nudges) to policy-based interventions, such as taxation on sugary beverages. Attitudes towards interventions based on choice architecture were also assessed in their study. In this case, respondents preferred interventions that were presented as effective in solving the problem, even when told about the automatic or 'System 1' nature of them. That is, generally speaking, as long as an intervention works, respondents rated them as acceptable even knowing that it works largely non-consciously.

BURNING ISSUE BOX 9.1

ARE NUDGES ETHICAL?

Some people might be uncomfortable with or even explicitly oppose nudges and choice architecture, especially if they are perceived as reducing personal autonomy and freedom, or if they are seen as 'sneaky' and being used outside of our awareness or consent. This issue is something that several researchers and economists (e.g., Fischer & Lotz, 2014) have discussed, under the broader consideration of the ethical implications of applying these principles, even if it is presumably for the 'greater good' of society.

One ethical concern with nudges is that nudging programs may actually exacerbate or contribute to health inequalities and disparities. Some communities simply have limited or no access to more optimal choices, like adequate health care and healthy food choices. This latter point is a concern in many parts of the world, including even in the US, where many rural regions are referred to as 'food deserts' because people in such regions (numbering about 23 million Americans) have no transportation and no supermarkets with fresh, healthy food within a mile. In the UK, food deserts (defined in the UK as being more than 500 meters from adequate food provisions) tend to be concentrated instead in urban areas (Wrigley, 2002). Choice architecture interventions are moot for such communities because the healthier options are not available in the first place. From this perspective, nudges and choice architecture can be seen as partially instrumental in perpetuating inequalities, such that those with privilege and access benefit from such interventions, and those without privilege and access cannot benefit from them in the first place.

Another ethical concern is that if nudging and choice architecture techniques are assumed to be effective and low-cost interventions, then other strategies (like economic and policy-based solutions, discussed below) might be abandoned. For example, instead of raising the price of tobacco or alcohol (economic policies which are known to be effective), there could be sole reliance on nudges to change behavior, which would be a mistake even if such nudges are perceived as being less paternalistic.

Sunstein (2015), one of the original co-authors of *Nudge*, has discussed the ethics of nudges in the light of several critiques, some of which are discussed above. Ethical arguments against nudges (see reviews in Kosters & Van der Heijden, 2015; see also Rachlin, 2015) are typically captured by the sentiment that our tendency to behave in certain default ways should not be used against us, such as increasing organ donation rates. This is especially true if such techniques are outside of our awareness or threaten our autonomy or our freedom to choose. Sunstein argues that nudges and choice architecture are everywhere already, and that they do not necessarily constrain human agency, but instead promote or facilitate it.

SOCIAL NORMS AS ENVIRONMENTAL GUIDES TO BEHAVIOR

There are two general types of social norms that guide behavior: descriptive and injunctive social norms. Descriptive norms refer simply to who is doing what, or to how many others are engaged in a certain behavior. For example, a perceived descriptive norm might include the percentage of university students that a particular person believes drinks lots of alcohol on regular occasions. These kinds of norms signal to us what is generally typical of those around us. Injunctive norms, on the other hand, refer to what others consider to be acceptable or unacceptable behavior. Perceived injunctive norms guide behavior by signaling what is acceptable, appropriate or valid behavior (Cialdini, Reno & Kallgren, 1990). They may also include sanctions or consequences for engaging in or refraining from certain behaviors. Descriptive and injunctive norms sometimes pull us in different directions. Jared may see many of his peers smoking cigarettes (descriptive norm), but he knows that his family and close friends would strongly disapprove (injunctive norm) if they were to discover him smoking.

In the UK in the last few years, there has been an embracing of these ideas by government in an attempt to address various public health behaviors that have social consequences. A Behavioral Insights Team was set up by the government in 2010 with the aim of using influence techniques like social norms and related concepts (discussed further below) to design simple interventions to change important behaviors. Concerning social norms, the Behavioral Insights Team has focused on the ways that healthy behaviors can spread contagiously through social networks. They cite a large study of American smokers and their families over three generations beginning in the late 1940s (Christakis & Fowler, 2008). In this study, people in close social networks exerted influence on each other, and it was observed that spouses and friends tended to quit smoking together. This is an example of how the behavior of other people can impact our own behavior.

INDIRECT IMPACTS ON BEHAVIOR: HOW CHANGING THE ENVIRONMENT MAY CHANGE COGNITIONS

While the social norms-type approach has features of direct environmental effects on behavior (i.e., that the effects are likely to work to a large extent relatively automatically), it is probable that this approach changes norms which in turn explains subsequent changes in behavior (i.e., a mediated approach).

The *social norms* approach has been used in attempts to change various behaviors, such as the misuse of alcohol and smoking initiation in young people (Haines, Barker & Rice, 2003). The key feature of this approach as a research tool is that individuals first provide information about their own behavior and attitudes. Later, the same individuals make estimates of the numbers of others in their local environment who perform the behavior or approve of the behavior. Feedback is then provided on the actual behaviors and attitudes of others based on the earlier survey. So, for example, an individual might estimate that about half the members of their school would approve of smoking and that about one quarter are actual smokers. Based on the survey they can then be provided with information to debunk these ideas by showing the actual numbers are quite a lot lower (e.g., showing that only 1 in 5 approve of smoking and only 1 in 10 actually smoke). The assumption is that this more accurate information concerning prevalent social norms will prompt the individuals to decide not to smoke and to be less likely to take up smoking in the future. There is some evidence for the success of this approach, particularly in relation to reducing drinking (Bewick et al., 2013; Moreira, Smith & Foxcroft, 2009). However, a recent review suggests that even medium-to-large changes in norms engender only small changes in drinking behavior and no change in alcohol-related problems (Prestwich et al., 2016). Other researchers (e.g., Chung, Christopoulos, King-Casas, Ball & Chiu, 2015; see also Smith & Delgado, 2015) have shown that exposure to others making either risky or safer decisions in domains like gambling or food choices influence the degree to which we make similar risky or safe decisions.

Burger and Shelton (2011) used a similar technique to change the use of stairs over the lift in order to promote physical activity. They found that a sign emphasizing the benefits of using the stairs only produced a modest increase in use of the stairs, while a sign emphasizing that most people used the stairs showed a significant increase in stair use (from 85% to 92% comparing before and after the sign).

In a meta-analytic review of several experimental tests of the effect of social norms on eating behavior, Robinson, Thomas, Aveyard and Higgs (2014) found clear evidence that informational social norms have an impact. When study participants were given a 'high intake norm,' or information about others consuming a lot of food, it increased the amount of food consumed, compared to control conditions. Likewise, the studies that manipulated a 'low intake norm' also found a significant effect such that, compared to controls, low intake norms reduced food consumption in study participants. In addition to impacting the quantity of food consumed, social norms can also impact the type of food chosen (healthy snacks versus junk food). It is worth nothing that in most of these studies (e.g., Cruwys et al., 2012; Robinson, Benwell & Higgs, 2013), participants are given free access to food such as popcorn, pizza or fruits and vegetables, so the dependent variables are objective, observable behaviors.

One caveat to the social norms approach, especially when considering *perceived* social norms, is that people often display a heuristic thinking pattern known as the False Consensus Effect, which means that they generally overestimate the prevalence of support for their attitudes, traits or behaviors (see Kenworthy & Miller, 2001; Krueger & Clement, 1994). In addition, there is evidence for a selective exposure effect in estimating agreement for our behavioral and attitudinal positions (e.g., Bosveld, Koomen & Pligt, 1994). This means that, when estimating the number of people who behave like us or share our opinions, we typically refer cognitively to those who are already similar to us to begin with. We might therefore believe that our unhealthy behaviors are more acceptable because of a perceived social norm that is artificially inflated due to heuristic thinking.

BURNING ISSUE BOX 9.2

HOW CAN INDIVIDUALS FOREGO PERSONAL GAINS FOR THE GREATER GOOD?

In 1968, Garrett Hardin published a paper in *Science* titled 'The Tragedy of the Commons.' This describes the story of how herdsmen add extra cows to their own herds for personal gains. Unfortunately, this ultimately destroys the communal land that the cows graze leading to hardship for all. Many environmental and health problems have a similar profile. In the short term, each individual wanting to travel in the city may gain by taking their car rather than using the bus (more convenience, comfort etc.). However, if everyone uses a car to travel, then in the longer term everyone will suffer due to poor air quality and increased traffic. In terms of public health, widespread immunization can help to break the chain of infection. However, in a population where a lot of people are immune there is a relatively low risk of infection anyway and there are drawbacks to the individual of being immunized (e.g., some people perceive certain immunizations to contain harmful ingredients, they have side effects etc.). By deciding to not vaccinate based on these assumptions, individuals risk the status of public immunity (as well as increasing their own risk for contracting harmful, infectious diseases); as the proportion of non-immune individuals increases in a population, the likelihood of disease outbreaks also increases (see Fu, Rosenbloom, Wang & Nowak, 2011).

Such a discussion is not just an academic exercise. In 2014, the Philippines had a severe outbreak of measles, and this disease was subsequently introduced to the US population. In that year, the US experienced 23 different measles outbreaks, infecting hundreds of people. The vast majority of those infected during these measles outbreaks were unvaccinated (Centers for Disease Control and Prevention, 2016). Mandatory immunization would help to protect the status of public immunity and solve the social dilemma, but there are some obvious ethical concerns with forced immunization. The good news is that general vaccination programs do work. Recently, the Americas were declared free of measles by the Pan American Health Organization, meaning that transmission of measles does not occur for local strains of the disease. The bad news is that strains from other countries can still be introduced to the Americas and infect non-vaccinated or susceptible people, and that decisions to not vaccinate are potentially a threat to public health.

Commons dilemmas can be difficult to resolve because the problem is not strongly influenced one way or another by a single individual taking action. One more person using the car rather than the bus will not markedly affect air pollution or congestion. Similarly, one person switching from using the car to the bus will have little impact in general. Indeed, for that individual, switching to traveling by bus in the city may not be in their interest (i.e., less comfort and flexibility). However, across a range of individual health behaviors, many individuals do choose to act in ways that might benefit the good of all to the potential detriment of their own perceived self-interests because individuals often consider the *right* or *moral* thing to do. According to the Norm Activation Model (NAM; Schwartz, 1977; Schwartz & Howard, 1984), a given behavior is adopted not because of the expected outcomes of performance, but for more internalized feelings that can be captured by the concept of moral or personal norm. Personal norms are activated when individuals are aware of the potential adverse consequences of their actions on others or on the environment, and when they believe they can reverse or prevent those consequences. Both sets of beliefs need to be made salient or applied for behavior consistent with the moral norm to occur and to actively influence behavior.

Returning to our example of car use contributing to air pollution, an individual needs to believe their car use is contributing to air pollution and that their reducing car use will help reduce air pollution before the moral norm will be activated (i.e., for the individual to decide it is the right thing to do to reduce use of their car and to take action). Schwartz (1977) proposed that these personal norms are not experienced as intentions, but as feelings of moral obligation and so can directly influence behavior rather than indirectly through changing intentions. A number of studies have shown the NAM to provide good levels of prediction of low-cost environmental behaviors like using public transport over personal cars. Others have argued that moral norms may also moderate the relationship between intentions and behavior by strengthening the relationship between intentions and behaviors perceived to have moral consequences (e.g., Godin, Conner & Sheeran, 2005).

One other aspect of the environment that has received quite a lot of research attention in terms of how its effects on behavior are mediated by other variables is *level of deprivation*. Deprivation can be measured in a number of ways including income, education and material deprivation (e.g., the extent to which the area you live in is materially deprived). Analyses of neighborhood-level indices of deprivation show that increasing deprivation is associated with lower levels of physical activity (see Cubbin et al., 2006; Sundquist, Malmstrom & Johansson, 1999).

In a sample of nearly 1,500 Canadian adults, Godin et al. (2010) examined level of education, family income, material deprivation and social deprivation as predictors of physical activity. Importantly, they also measured intention and perceived behavioral control (PBC) over physical activity in the same sample. This was done to allow for tests of mediation effects on subsequent physical activity. In their data, simple correlations showed education, income and material deprivation to be significantly associated with physical activity levels (social deprivation was not significantly associated with physical activity levels). As you might guess, physical activity was higher among those who were better educated, had higher income and were less deprived. However, these effects were modest compared to the effects for intention and PBC. Specifically, the effect sizes for the environmental variables were small, but the effect sizes for intentions and PBC were of medium magnitude. Interestingly, the effects of both education and income were partially mediated by intention and PBC (there were no significant effects for material deprivation). These findings suggest that part, but not all, of the effect of education and income on physical activity is explained by differences in intentions and PBC for physical activity. In other words, having less education and/or less income results in lower levels of engaging in physical activity partly *because* education and income also yield lower levels of intention and PBC over physical activity. The fact that mediation is partial in this case suggests there are likely other mechanisms by which education and income impact on physical activity levels. For example, it may be the case that such people have fewer opportunities to be physically active in sports centers.

Getting a better understanding of when cognitions do not mediate, partially mediate or completely mediate the effects of changes in the environment on behavior might help us design more effective interventions. For example, where the effects of the environment are mediated by cognitions, it may be useful to consider combining interventions that target environmental changes (e.g., providing more sports centers) with ones that target different cognition changes (e.g., strengthening intentions to be physically active).

HOW THE ENVIRONMENT INTERACTS WITH COGNITIONS IN DETERMINING BEHAVIOR

In addition to mediated effects, we may also find **moderated effects**, or interaction effects, between aspects of the environment and cognitions about the behavior itself, in determining behavior. In general, an interaction effect means that the direct effect of one variable, such as the environment, is different for different groups of people. These groups may be based on experimental conditions, created by random assignment, or they may be formed by self-selection, such as when people prefer to live in one neighborhood over another because of factors such as income, ethnicity or religion. Comparisons of differential effects can also use groups based on individual differences or personality factors. For example, the influence of intentions to engage in healthy behaviors on actual behavior might be strongest for people who score high on personality-level conscientiousness.

The study by Godin et al. (2010) that we considered above contains one example of such an interactive, or moderated, effect. Godin et al. showed that, in addition to the mediation of intentions and PBC on behavior, education level *moderated* the effect of intentions to engage in physical activity on subsequent physical activity levels: intentions were weaker predictors of physical activity among the less educated participants than among the more educated. This is quite important because it suggests that interventions designed to increase intentions to engage in physical activity in a sample or population (as is common in many health promotion messages) will be less effective for those with less education compared to those with more education. It could be the case that among those with less education an intervention targeting intentions to engage in physical activity needs to also target some of the tangible barriers to physical activity.

Concerning health behaviors generally, a key environmental variable has been **socio-economic status (SES)**. SES refers to the social standing of an individual or group in the social hierarchy, and is measured by factors such as relative material deprivation, income, education and occupational classification. Low SES is consistently associated with both increased morbidity and mortality rates (Adler et al., 1994; Centers for Disease Control and Prevention, 2011). In addition, research has demonstrated parallel differences in engagement with a variety of health behaviors as a function of SES (Blaxter, 1990; Ford et al., 1991). For example, health risk behaviors such as smoking and alcohol dependency tend to be higher for low SES groups compared to high SES groups, and health protective behaviors such as physical activity and healthy eating tend to be lower. In fact, recent research has suggested the link between SES and mortality is attributable to differences in engagement with various health behaviors (Nandi, Glymour & Subramanian, 2014; Stringhini et al., 2010).

One pertinent question is whether SES also moderates the effects of *cognitions* on health behaviors. Findings from Conner et al. (2013) suggest this to be the case. They found that the relationship between intentions to engage in a specific health behavior and subsequent performance was moderated by participants' level of SES: lower SES weakened the intention-behavior relationship.

Other types of moderation effects have been detected. For example, O'Brien (2012), using a longitudinal design of US adults over 10 years, found that SES (operationalized as the number of years of education) was (as expected) a strong predictor of changes in chronic illness (including diabetes, lupus, cancer etc.) over time, such that less educated respondents reported significantly greater increases in chronic illnesses. However, control beliefs (including both personal mastery and personal constraints/obstacles) interacted with SES in predicting changes in reported chronic illness. When control beliefs were weak, there was a significant difference between low SES and high SES respondents. However, when control beliefs were strong, no differences were found between low and high SES groups. Another way to look at their findings is to consider that the greatest increases in chronic illness were reported among respondents with both low SES and weak control beliefs.

POLICY-BASED APPROACHES TO BEHAVIOR CHANGE

In relation to policy-based approaches to behavior change we will now examine how making behaviors illegal (e.g., seat belt wearing), changing pricing (e.g., for alcohol and tobacco, high sugar drinks) and requiring health warnings (e.g., fat consumption, texting and driving, smoking) have been shown to be effective means of changing a range of health behaviors. In this section we will discuss findings based on examining the direct behavioral outcomes of public policies, and we will also discuss a subset or corollary of the policy-based approach, which is typically referred to as the *social marketing* approach to behavior change.

The approaches that fall under the category of policy-based interventions are generally of two types. They will either be based on an informational strategy, or be based on changing the market environment itself. Informational approaches are focused on getting people to think more about their choices, or to be aware of the benefits of certain choices or the dangers of other choices (see also the 'empowerment' approach; Feufel et al., 2011). One drawback to these approaches is that they may not reliably result in behavior change even though people may be more knowledgeable, aware or persuaded about the consequences of certain behaviors. The other type of strategy involves changing the market environment directly. These may be seen as more difficult, expensive and intrusive (see Brambila-Macias et al., 2011), but tend to be quite effective in producing changes to behavior and other desired psychological outcomes. In this section, we will review some important areas of health behavior where changes to policies have had measureable impacts.

SEAT BELTS

Over the past few decades the mandatory use of seat belts in motor vehicles has increased to the point where most developed countries now have compulsory seat belt laws. There are variations to these laws, both across countries as well as within them. In the US, for example, each state has its own seat belt laws. Currently, the only US state without compulsory seat belts for adults is New Hampshire, whose state motto is, appropriately, 'Live Free or Die.'

The introduction of seat belt laws has reduced fatalities and related outcomes in the UK (Rutherford, 1985) and the US (Cohen & Einav, 2003). It is unclear, however, what psychological mechanisms might be at work generally in producing greater compliance with seat belt laws. It could be the case that seat belt laws have a direct effect on behavior. Alternatively, such laws may change cognitive processes, which in turn affect behavior. For example, Stasson and Fishbein (1990) reported that perceived risk (of injury/death) does not have a direct effect on seat belt usage. Instead, that behavior is predicted proximally by intentions to use a seat belt. In their study, intentions were best predicted by perceived risk and social norms. Sutton and Eiser (1990) also showed that fear arousal and perceived risk predicted seat belt use intentions, but that over time intentions became less important and past behavior (i.e., automatic tendencies, or habits)

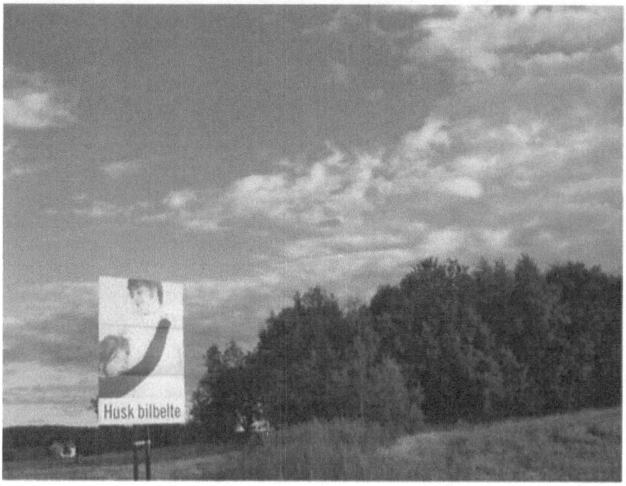

FIGURE 9.2 This Norwegian advertisement emphasizes important social connections to remind people to wear their seat belts while driving

emerged as the main predictor of seat belt use. Regardless of the exact mechanisms, policies and laws requiring the use of seat belts increase seat belt usage and ultimately prevent injuries and save lives.

TEXTING AND DRIVING

In the UK, using a handheld device while driving has been illegal since 2003, but of the UK vehicle fatalities caused by distractions in 2012, nearly 20% of those were due to mobile phone usage. Although there are not (yet) many long-term studies examining the effectiveness of mobile phone restrictions, there are some recently published articles that shed some light on the issue. One such study (Ehsani, Bingham, Ionides & Childers, 2014; see also Highway Loss Data Institute, 2010) reported an increase in crashes following the introduction of a 2010 texting restriction law put into place in the US state of Michigan. Ehsani et al. speculate that this result may be due to an unintended consequence of the law, which is that people will likely deliberately conceal their mobile phone use behavior while driving so as to avoid being seen by others, especially by police officers/law enforcement. Thus, by keeping their mobile phones out of sight, their driving vision impairments and distractions are exacerbated.

However, larger-scale studies tell a different story. Ferdinand et al. (2014; see also Abouk & Adams, 2013) used a specialized vehicle fatality reporting system to examine the rate of fatal vehicle accidents across 10 years in the US, comparing states with and without texting restrictions or bans. They found a difference overall in fatalities between states with primary bans on texting (drivers can be stopped and fined because they are using their mobile phones), compared to states with secondary bans (drivers must be stopped for some other infraction first, then may be issued a fine for mobile phone usage). Specifically, secondary bans on texting had no effect on traffic fatalities, whereas primary bans did have an effect on reducing fatalities. In fact, the primary bans were found to have the strongest life-saving impact on the sector of the population most at-risk for texting-related accidents and deaths: young people.

Thus, generally speaking, although mobile phone use bans may produce a shift in behavior from overt to covert in some cases, such laws do have a positive effect on reducing accidents and on saving lives. However, researchers should examine the social and cognitive mechanisms by which better, less distracted driving behavior can be encouraged.

DRINK DRIVING

There are various policies, laws and blood alcohol content (BAC) limits in countries around the world, some of which are much more stringent than others. These limits range from an upper limit of around 0.08% (e.g., Mexico, US, Canada) down to 0% (e.g., Brazil, Czech Republic, United Arab Emirates). There are also variations in these laws within countries, such as more stringent restrictions on younger drivers or on commercial operators. The penalties for drink driving offenses also vary widely. In the state of California, for example, a new law will go into effect in 2019, requiring that all first-time offenders install an ignition-lock breathalyzer in their vehicle or else be restricted to driving only to and from work or on other necessary trips.

Because drink driving has been a serious public health problem for a long time, a variety of policy- and law-based solutions have been tested and implemented over the years. For example, Fell and Voas (2006) examined the outcomes of 14 different studies on the effectiveness of BAC-limit laws, around the US and in Europe and Australia, and concluded that having lower BAC limits (e.g., from 0.08% to 0.05% or lower) does serve to reduce the number of vehicle accidents, injuries and deaths. Some of the more effective laws, apart from BAC laws described above, include license bans/suspension, publicized sobriety checkpoints, alcohol ignition locks (for repeat offenders), minimum drinking age laws and zero tolerance laws (see Goodwin et al., 2015).

WARNING LABELS AND PRICE HIKES

Over the years, there have been many tests of the question of whether price or tax increases on certain products have their desired effects. Bader, Boisclair and Ferrence (2011) reviewed many such studies in relation to smoking and found that the majority of studies reviewed did find that increasing the price of tobacco products reduced both the prevalence of youth smoking behavior as well as the amount of tobacco that they consumed. The evidence is more mixed concerning the initiation or uptake of smoking behavior, however; some studies found some impact on preventing smoking, whereas others found no effect at all. One concern with raising prices or taxes on certain products is that such a policy risks being socially regressive, or more punishing to the finances of poorer people. That is, they must spend a greater proportion of their total income on raised prices, compared to wealthier people. Thus, Bader et al. examined whether price increases on tobacco products had differential effects on low SES versus higher SES groups of consumers. Although a minority of studies reviewed showed that increasing tobacco prices is good for all socioeconomic groups approximately equally as far as the reduction in smoking participation and consumption are concerned, the majority of studies reviewed showed an equal or better impact of price increases on low SES groups compared to the general population. Specifically, increasing tobacco prices is good for all socioeconomic groups approximately equally as far as the reduction in smoking participation and consumption are concerned. However, one of the unintended consequences of price increases is that lower SES groups tend to show more demand for smuggled cigarettes when prices go up (e.g., Thomas et al., 2008; Wiltshire, Bancroft, Amos & Parry, 2001).

TOBACCO AND SUGARY DRINKS

With taxes and price hikes on sugared products being implemented in both the UK and in the US, the key question of course is whether and how they work in favor of public health. Researchers in both countries (e.g., Brownell & Frieden, 2009; Michie, 2016) argue for a tax on sugar-sweetened beverages because such a policy would almost certainly improve health and reduce obesity. Such beverages are seen as a leading cause of obesity, and reductions in sugar beverage intake are clearly associated with improved health over time (see Vartanian, Schwartz & Brownell, 2007). One point of uncertainty in this research so far concerns which alternative foods people would buy instead of sugary drinks. Cartwright (2014) argues that warning label policies are good for academics and people who think rationally about the relationships among consumption of calories, weight gain and associated diseases. However, warning labels are perhaps unlikely to have much of an impact on people who struggle with weight gain for a variety of reasons. One of the ethical considerations for warning labels about obesity is that such labels may lead to further stigmatization and moral judgment of people who choose to consume such products.

Concerning the issue of the effectiveness of warning labels on behavioral choice, VanEpps and Roberto (2016) conducted a representative online study to test whether warning labels for sugar-sweetened beverages can influence beverage choices. They gathered responses from over 2,200 adolescents aged 12–18 years. The key independent variable was the type of label accompanying different drinks. They compared a condition with no warning label to a condition with just a calorie indicator label, and to four different types of health warnings telling the prospective consumer that sugary drinks were linked to weight gain, obesity, diabetes and tooth decay. The main outcome in this study was a hypothetical choice of beverage from a vending machine. Warning labels, compared to control and calorie-only labels, generally and significantly reduced the percentage of participants choosing sugar-sweetened beverages.

Because increasing taxes on sugary drinks is such a recent phenomenon, there is relatively little data so far concerning the actual behavioral purchasing habits of consumers, not to mention the longer-term health effects of such policies. Some recent findings are encouraging, however. In California, voters in two neighboring cities (San Francisco and Berkeley) voted in 2014 on proposals to add a sugar tax to beverages sold in those cities (see Charles, 2016). Voters in Berkeley approved the tax, whereas voters in San Francisco rejected the proposal. This 'natural experiment' yielded some important, if preliminary data. Compared to baseline data, in which residents in both cities reported drinking about 1.5 sugary, fizzy drinks per day, the sugar tax seems to have had its intended effects. Residents in Berkeley reported about 20% lower consumption

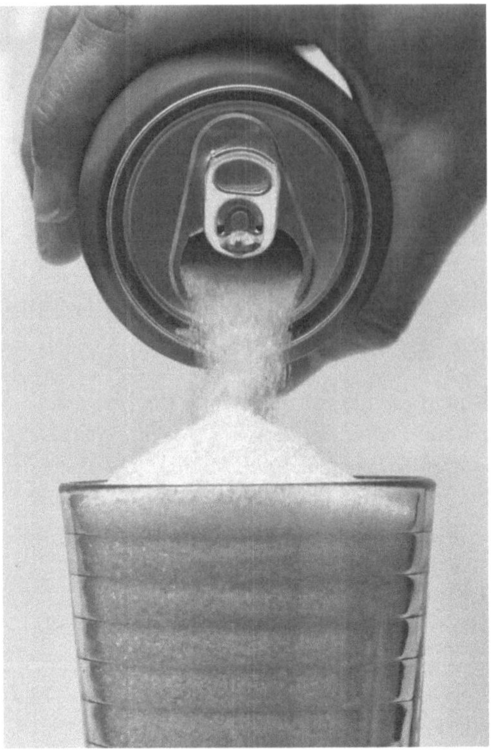

FIGURE 9.3 Most 12-ounce sugary drinks contain about 10 teaspoons of sugar!

of sugary drinks (and an increase in reported water consumption) following the introduction of the tax, whereas reported consumption of sugary drinks in San Francisco did not change over time. Of course, it remains to be seen whether such taxes in the UK and the US have their desired effects on behavior and health over the long term, not just on raising money for government programs. One recent meta-analysis provides some information on this issue. Cabrera Escobar, Veerman, Tollman, Bertram and Hofman (2013) gathered studies from around the world (e.g., Brazil, France, Mexico, USA) in which the authors examined the effects of price hikes or taxes on sugar-sweetened beverages, and found that such policies do tend to reduce obesity and BMI, and that they may be effective policies generally, despite their 'regressive' nature. There is no doubt that many researchers will continue to collect data on this issue in order to understand not just what the patterns of behavior are, but why and under what conditions they occur.

SOCIAL MARKETING APPROACH TO BEHAVIOR CHANGE

As an increasingly popular method of health promotion, social marketing tries to influence behavior by offering people tangible and social benefits, by reducing barriers and constraints that may block them physically or emotionally, and by using persuasion in targeted or personalized ways to create behavior change. It is a model that differs from traditional health promotion programs, which tend to simply instruct people on how to behave. Instead, social marketing is about getting people to 'buy' the better behavior because it is desirable and worth their time, energy or resources (Grier & Bryant, 2005).

The core of the social marketing approach is applying known and proven techniques of influence in consumer behavior to encourage or promote change in health behaviors (see Andreasen, 2002). The ideal outcome is that individuals make more healthy choices for their own benefit as well for the benefit of society as a whole (Luca & Suggs, 2013; Spotswood, French, Tapp & Stead, 2012). According to this approach, researchers and practitioners should examine and understand the values and beliefs that motivate and underlie a variety of health behaviors, so that those values and beliefs can be targeted in creating messages or interventions that have the greatest likelihood of effecting change. Although you will undoubtedly recognize this as similar to other models and theories discussed in this book so far, proponents of the social marketing approach argue that it is distinct in some key ways.

According to Andreasen (2002), there are six criteria that should be met in order for an intervention to qualify as social marketing. First, the intervention must focus on behavior change (rather than intentions or attitudes) in its design and evaluation. Second, social marketing should focus on the motives and needs of the target audience, including both pretesting ideas and monitoring them as they are implemented. Third, interventions should be tailored to specific segments of the population (e.g., based on ethnicity, sex, language etc.), without assuming that a general intervention can be implemented for all members of a population. Fourth, the intervention should be based on exchange theory, emphasizing the rewards of behavior change and lowering the costs of compliance. Fifth, the intervention should utilize the four Ps of traditional marketing: *Product* (rewards, benefits), *Price* (cost, effort), *Place* (ease of access) and *Promotion* (relevance to the target audience). Finally, the intervention should be designed around an understanding of the competition for an individual's behavior change choices. That is, the behavior change strategy should focus on minimizing the likelihood of other possible behaviors, including current behaviors.

Social marketing strategies and interventions have been developed and used in a variety of countries and cultures, and for an array of health behaviors. One innovative program utilizing this approach was designed to increase the use of insecticide-treated mosquito nets in Tanzania (Kikumbih, Hanson, Mills, Mponda & Schellenberg, 2005) through social promotion of this behavior using stickers, flags, shirts and billboards. The campaign increased the usage of mosquito nets in the intervention area, compared to a control area of the country.

In a social marketing campaign involving nearly 3,000 Canadian university students, Scarapicchia et al. (2015) aimed to increase self-efficacy, outcome expectancies, behavioral intentions to exercise and, ultimately, changes in moderate to vigorous physical activity. You probably recognize these constructs from the theories discussed in earlier chapters. Their campaign contained social marketing elements emphasizing the benefits of exercise, including stress reduction, enjoyment and academic achievement. These messages were disseminated in postcards, posters, online social media, in classrooms and via face-to-face interactions with peer 'ambassadors' from the campaign. Overall, their findings supported the model that they proposed based on the social marketing principles as well as the theoretical framework guiding the choice of measured variables. Specifically, awareness of the campaign predicted greater outcome expectancies (e.g., 'Regular physical activity helps me manage stress'), which were associated with greater perceived self-efficacy (e.g., 'I am confident that I can regularly do 30 minutes or more of moderate physical activity per day most days of the week'). In turn self-efficacy predicted both stronger intentions to be physically active as well as higher self-reported participation in moderate and vigorous physical activity.

In addition to a focus on increasing healthy behaviors, several studies aim to reduce or prevent harmful behaviors. Glider, Midyett, Mills-Novoa, Johannessen and Collins (2001), using a social marketing intervention that included school newspaper advertisements, awareness activities and interviews in the local radio and television media, reduced alcohol-related behaviors within the university population. They also saw changes in perceived campus norms, including a significant decrease in the percentage of students who believe that most students have five or more drinks at parties, and that drinking alcohol makes sexual opportunities more likely. However, the study was limited as it did not employ a control group.

Rather than the mediated-type effect demonstrated by Glider et al., a similar intervention conducted in Australia found a moderated effect. In this study, Dietrich et al. (2015) randomly assigned 20 high schools to an alcohol social marketing intervention and another 20 schools to serve as no-exposure controls and found differential effects of social marketing across different segments of the population studied: abstainers, bingers and moderate drinkers. For example, participation in the intervention resulted in a significant reduction in intentions to binge drink, but only among the bingers. For them, their changed knowledge about, and attitudes towards drinking impacted their subsequent intentions to binge drink. The same pattern was not observed for the abstainers and moderate drinkers, but their baseline intentions to binge drink were already quite low to begin with.

In an early review of social marketing interventions, Gordon, McDermott, Stead and Angus (2006) found the approach to be effective in increasing consumption of fruits and vegetables, reducing fat intake and improving people's attitudes towards healthy eating; the findings were more heterogeneous for physical activity, with several studies showing a positive effect on exercise and several showing no effects (but was seemingly effective for changing people's awareness, knowledge or attitudes about exercise); and reasonably successful for substance misuse such as smoking and illicit drug use (although social marketing was less effective in smoking cessation than in preventing or reducing smoking behavior). Gordon et al. also report that social marketing interventions can be effective across a range of different target groups and in different settings, such as in schools, churches, workplaces and even in supermarkets.

Limitations to the social marketing approach

There are a number of limitations to this approach. First, Kubacki, Rundle-Thiele, Pang and Buyucek (2015) noted that, despite a focus in the literature on six key, benchmark criteria (discussed above; see Andreasen, 2002) of a social marketing intervention, few studies employ all six criteria.

Second, some critics (e.g., Langford & Panter-Brick, 2013) argue that social marketing focuses too much on individual agency and individual behavior, without taking into account the very real structural constraints of many populations, especially disadvantaged populations that are often the most in need of health interventions. For example, when individuals in disadvantaged populations or areas become motivated to change via social marketing campaigns, they often cannot because of resource constraints. In the end, they may have even worse outcomes because they can feel powerless to act, and ashamed or stigmatized for not changing their behavior.

Third, and as a related point, because many of the principal factors influencing health behavior are social and political, public health campaigns (including those using social marketing) should include attempts to change public policy so that the barriers and constraints on opportunities can be reduced or removed for everyone. Such a sentiment is not inconsistent with the major theorist, integrated model of behavior change presented elsewhere in this book, in which constraints are a major factor in determining behavior change.

Fourth, although the studies testing social marketing can possess good external validity, they tend to suffer from a lack of internal validity. Such studies employ their methods in the real world, outside of the laboratory, so they cannot typically randomly assign their participants to conditions or get representative, random samples of their populations. Caution is warranted because these approaches tend to combine several variables or interventions together, and they lack strong theoretical frameworks. This makes it difficult for scientists and consumers to have a clear sense of which factors are responsible for any observed effects, or of why they occurred in the first place. On the other hand, applying techniques in a problem-focused way is often done with the goal of solving some social problem – in this case improving individual and public health. Thus, we may see a sacrificing of strict internal validity to research when lives are at stake.

Finally, if these strategies are seen to be effective, then they will likely require long-term investments by communities and their respective governments. This is because such interventions must compete against a constant array of countervailing forces encouraging us to engage in unhealthy behaviors.

SCIENCE OF HEALTH BEHAVIOR CHANGE: IN ACTION

In Action Box 9.1 considers an experiment by Robinson et al. (2013). In this study, the authors examined the impact of different social norms on eating behavior. They manipulated a low intake norm, a high intake norm and a no norm control condition, and measured how many cookies participants ate following the presentation of those norms. The theory suggests that such norms will act as direct modeling influences on eating behavior, so the authors expected that participants would eat more cookies than controls in the high intake norm condition, and fewer cookies than controls in the low intake norm condition.

SCIENCE OF HEALTH BEHAVIOR CHANGE

In Action Box 9.1

Study: Robinson et al. (2013). *Food intake norms increase and decrease snack food intake in a remote confederate study*

Aim: To examine the effects of social norms on snack food intake.

Method: Participants were randomized to one of three conditions: a low intake norm, a high intake norm and no norm (control). Under the cover story of a taste test, they were presented with a well-stocked bowl of cookies, and were left alone to eat for 15 minutes. Empathy levels were also measured; this variable was expected to predict the outcomes as well.

Results: The intake norms affected behavior as expected, such that participants consumed the fewest number of cookies in the low intake norm condition, the highest number of cookies in the high intake norm condition and an intermediate number in the control condition. Empathy had no direct or interactive effect on eating behavior.

Authors' conclusion: Participants given intake norms from (fictitious) prior participants matched those norms in their own eating behavior. Social norms for eating can have a strong influence on eating behavior.

THEORY AND TECHNIQUES OF HEALTH BEHAVIOR CHANGE		
BCTs	INTERVENTION: Based on Michie et al.'s (2013) taxonomy: Low intake and high intake norm conditions: 6.2 Social comparison.	
	CONTROL: None	
Critical Skills Toolkit		
3.1	Does the design enable the identification of which BCTs are effective?	*Yes – the intervention manipulates norms only (which in the Michie et al., 2013, taxonomy is labeled social comparison).*
4.1	Is the intervention based on one theory or a combination of theories (if any at all)?	*The intervention is based on the findings of previous studies but no formal theory is explicitly noted as providing the basis for the intervention.*
	Are all constructs specified within a theory targeted by the intervention?	*Not applicable – no formal theory stated.*
	Are all behavior change techniques explicitly targeting at least one theory-relevant construct?	*Not applicable – no formal theory stated.*
	Do the authors test why the intervention was effective or ineffective (consistent with the underlying theory)?	*No; mediation analyses were not conducted.*
4.2	Does the study tailor the intervention based on the underlying theory?	*Not applicable – no formal theory stated.*

2.1, 2.2	What are the strengths/limitations of the underlying theory?	*Not applicable – no formal theory stated.*
	THE METHODOLOGY OF HEALTH BEHAVIOR CHANGE	
5.1, 5.3, 5.4, 5.6	Methodological approach	*The study adopted an experimental design (see Critical Skills Toolkit 5.4).*
6.1	For experimental designs: is the study between-subjects, within-subjects or mixed?	*Participants were allocated to one of three conditions (between-subjects) and completed key measures (eating) at a single time-point. For advantages and disadvantages of this design, see Critical Skills Toolkit 6.1.*
5.2, 5.5	Are the measures reliable and valid?	*The main outcome variable – eating cookies – was measured objectively.*
5.5	May other variables have been manipulated other than the independent variable?	*Low risk of bias. The manipulations appeared appropriate. Thus, the internal validity of the experiment was not threatened by the risk of confounds.*
	Non-random allocation of participants to condition	*Low risk. Participants were randomized to conditions, and did not differ across groups on baseline hunger, fullness, desire to eat or BMI.*
	Blinding and allocation concealment	*Unclear risk. There was no evidence of blinding or allocation concealment in the procedure.* *There was also some risk of demand effects given the presentation of previous participants' eating behavior.*
	ANALYZING HEALTH BEHAVIOR CHANGE DATA	
6.2	Was the sample size calculated a-priori?	*The sample size was not calculated a-priori.*
Fig. 6.1	Was the hypothesis tested with an appropriate statistical test?	*Yes.*
5.5, 6.4	Incomplete outcome data	*Results were presented with the removal of two participants – one who guessed the aims of the study, and one who failed the manipulation check. The impact of removing these participants from the analyses was not reported.*
5.5	Selective outcome reporting	*Unclear given the trial protocol was not pre-published – however, all of the measures reported in the Method section were analyzed and reported in the Results section.*

4.2	Lack of variability (non-sig. effects only)	*Empathy was measured, but it did not affect the outcomes, either as a main effect or as an interaction with intake norm condition. However, there was no indication that there was a lack of variability on this measure across the sample.*
6.3	Non-linear relationship (non-sig. effects only)	*Non-linear effects were not tested.*

SUMMARY

In the first part of this chapter, we examined some direct environmental factors that influence behavior, including positive reinforcements, nudging and choice architecture interventions. We then explored some indirect or mediated effects of the environment on health behavior, such as when environmental factors lead to changes in cognition, which in turn affect behavior. Interactive or moderated effects were then examined, including when the effects of environmental factors are different depending on the type or group of persons in question. In the second part of the chapter, we explored a series of policy-based approaches to changing behavior, followed by a consideration of the social marketing approach to behavior change.

FURTHER READING

French, J. & Gordon, R. (2015). *Strategic Social Marketing.* London: Sage. This popular book introduces and critically evaluates the value of the social marketing approach to changing behavior and solving social problems.

Hardin, G. (1968). The tragedy of the commons. *Science, 162*, 1243–1248. This philosophical paper is an early introduction to the social dilemma of freedom of choice when resources are limited.

Kahneman, D. (2011). *Thinking, Fast and Slow.* New York: Farrar, Straus, and Giroux. Nobel Prize winner Daniel Kahneman uses his decades of experience in the psychology of decision-making to explore the various influences on our choices. Includes a discussion of System 1 and System 2 thinking.

Thaler, R. & Sunstein, C. (2008). *Nudge: Improving Decisions about Health, Wealth and Happiness.* London: Penguin. *Nudge* is easy and amusing to read, but deals with the serious topic of decision-making and its consequences in the real world.

Van Vugt, M. (2009). Averting the tragedy of the commons: using social psychological science to protect the environment. *Current Directions in Psychological Science, 18*, 169–173. Van Vugt summarizes relevant empirical evidence from social psychology, and makes some recommendations and predictions for research to address environmental behavior.

GLOSSARY

Choice architecture: part of Nudge Theory, suggesting that we can alter the environment in which decisions are made to make certain choices more or less likely.

Direct effect: simple case where changes in behavior are explained by changes in the environment.

Indirect/mediated effect: where changes in behavior are explained by changes in the ways that individuals view the behavior, such as cognitions about the environment, which in turn are caused by changes in the environment.

Moderated effect: where the relationship between cognitions and behavior is explained by changes in the environment (e.g., living in a deprived area reducing the impact of your intentions to not smoke on your subsequent smoking behavior).

Socio-economic status (SES): refers to the social standing of an individual or group in a social hierarchy and is measured by factors such as relative material deprivation, income, education and occupational classification.

System 1 thinking: refers to non-reflective, automatic or impulsive influences on behavior.

System 2 thinking: refers to more effortful, conscious, deliberative and reflective thought processes impacting behavior.

REFERENCES

Abouk, R. & Adams, S. (2013). Texting bans and fatal accidents on roadways: do they work? Or do drivers just react to announcements of bans? *American Economic Journal: Applied Economics*, *5*(2), 179–199.

Adler, N.E., Boyce, T., Chesney, M.A., Cohen, S., Folkman, S., Kahn, R.L. et al. (1994). Socioeconomic status and health. The challenge of the gradient. *American Psychologist*, *49*, 15–24.

Ajzen, I. (1991). The theory of planned behavior. *Organizational Behavior and Human Decision Processes*, *50*, 179–211.

Andreasen, A.R. (2002). Marketing social marketing in the social change marketplace. *Journal of Public Policy & Marketing*, *21*(1), 3–13.

Bader, P., Boisclair, D. & Ferrence, R. (2011). Effects of tobacco taxation and pricing on smoking behavior in high-risk populations: a knowledge synthesis. *International Journal of Environmental Research and Public Health*, *8*(11), 4118–4139.

Bewick, B.M., Bell, D., Crosby, S., Edlin, B., Keenan, S., Marshall, K. & Savva, G. (2013). Promoting improvements in public health: using a Social Norms Approach to reduce use of alcohol, tobacco and other drugs. *Drugs: Education, Prevention and Policy*, *20*(4), 322–330. doi: 10.3109/09687637.2013.766150.

Blaxter, M. (1990). *Health and Lifestyles*. London: Tavistock.

Bosveld, W., Koomen, W. & Pligt, J. (1994). Selective exposure and the false consensus effect: the availability of similar and dissimilar others. *British Journal of Social Psychology*, *33*(4), 457–466.

Brambila-Macias, J., Shankar, B., Capacci, S., Mazzocchi, M., Perez-Cueto, F.J., Verbeke, W. & Traill, W.B. (2011). Policy interventions to promote healthy eating: a review of what works, what does not, and what is promising. *Food and Nutrition Bulletin*, *32*(4), 365–375.

Brownell, K.D. & Frieden, T.R. (2009). Ounces of prevention – the public policy case for taxes on sugared beverages. *New England Journal of Medicine*, *360*(18), 1805–1808.

Burger, J.M. & Shelton, M. (2011). Changing everyday health behaviours through descriptive norm manipulations. *Social Influence, 6*, 69–77.

Cabrera Escobar, M.A., Veerman, J.L., Tollman, S.M., Bertram, M.Y. & Hofman, K.J. (2013). Evidence that a tax on sugar sweetened beverages reduces the obesity rate: a meta-analysis. *BMC Public Health, 13*, 1072. doi.org/10.1186/1471–2458–13–1072.

Cartwright, M.M. (2014). *Soda Warning Labels: Rated 'F' for Futility: Why Warning Labels on Sugary Beverages Will Not Impact Obesity*. Retrieved on June 30, 2017 from: www.psychologytoday.com/blog/food-thought/201406/soda-warning-labels-rated-f-futility-0

Centers for Diseases Control and Prevention. (2011). CDC health disparities and inequalities report – United States, 2011. *Morbidity and Mortality Weekly Reports, 60*, 1–113.

Centers for Diseases Control and Prevention. (2016). *Measles Cases and Outbreaks*. Retrieved on September 30, 2016 from: www.cdc.gov/measles/cases-outbreaks.html.

Charles, D. (2016). *Berkeley's Soda Tax Appears To Cut Consumption Of Sugary Drinks*. Retrieved on June 30, 2017 from: www.npr.org/sections/thesalt/2016/08/23/491104093/berkeleys-soda-tax-appears-to-cut-consumption-of-sugary-drinks.

Christakis, N.A. & Fowler, J.H. (2008) The collective dynamics of smoking in a large social network. *New England Journal of Medicine, 358*(21), 2249–2258.

Chung, D., Christopoulos, G.I., King-Casas, B., Ball, S.B. & Chiu, P.H. (2015). Social signals of safety and risk confer utility and have asymmetric effects on observers' choices. *Nature Neuroscience, 18*(6), 912–916.

Cialdini, R.B., Reno, R.R. & Kallgren, C.A. (1990). A focus theory of normative conduct: recycling the concept of norms to reduce littering in public places. *Journal of Personality and Social Psychology, 58*, 1015–1026.

Cohen, A. & Einav, L. (2003). The effects of mandatory seat belt laws on driving behavior and traffic fatalities. *Review of Economics and Statistics, 85*(4), 828–843.

Conner, M., McEachan, R., Jackson, C., McMillan, B., Woolridge, M. & Lawton, R. (2013). Moderating effect of socioeconomic status on the relationship between health cognitions and behaviors. *Annals of Behavioral Medicine, 46*(1), 19–30.

Cruwys, T., Platow, M.J., Angullia, S.A., Chang, J.M., Diler, S.E. Kirchner, J.L., ... & Wadley, A.L. (2012). Modeling of food intake is moderated by salient psychological group membership. *Appetite, 58*(2), 754–757.

Cubbin, C., Sundquist, K., Ahlen, H., Johansson, S.E., Winkleby, M.A. & Sundquist, J. (2006). Neighborhood deprivation and cardiovascular disease risk factors: protective and harmful effects. *Scandinavian Journal of Public Health, 34*, 228–237.

Dietrich, T., Rundle-Thiele, S., Schuster, L., Drennan, J., Russell-Bennett, R., Leo, C., ... & Connor, J.P. (2015). Differential segmentation responses to an alcohol social marketing program. *Addictive Behaviors, 49*, 68–77.

Ehsani, J.P., Bingham, C.R., Ionides, E. & Childers, D. (2014). The impact of Michigan's text messaging restriction on motor vehicle crashes. *Journal of Adolescent Health, 54*(5), S68–S74.

Faith, M.S., Rose, E., Matz, P.E., Pietrobelli, A. & Epstein, L.H. (2006). Co-twin control designs for testing behavioral economic theories of child nutrition: methodological note. *International Journal of Obesity, 30*(10), 1501–1505.

Fell, J.C. & Voas, R.B. (2006). The effectiveness of reducing illegal blood alcohol concentration (BAC) limits for driving: evidence for lowering the limit to .05 BAC. *Journal of Safety Research, 37*(3), 233–243.

Ferdinand, A.O., Menachemi, N., Sen, B., Blackburn, J.L., Morrisey, M. & Nelson, L. (2014). Impact of texting laws on motor vehicular fatalities in the United States. *American Journal of Public Health, 104*(8), 1370–1377.

Feufel, M.A., Antes, G., Steurer, J., Gigerenzer, G., Muir Gray, J.A., Mäkelä, M., ... & Wennberg, J.E. (2011). How to achieve better health care: better systems, better patients, or both? In G. Gigerenzer & J.A.M. Gray (Eds.), *Better Doctors, Better Patients, Better Decisions: Envisioning Healthcare 2020* (pp. 117–134). Cambridge, MA: MIT Press.

Fischer, M. & Lotz, S. (2014). Is soft paternalism ethically legitimate? – The relevance of psychological processes for the assessment of nudge-based policies. *Cologne Graduate School Working Paper Series (05–02)*. Retrieved on May 30, 2014 from: https://ideas.repec.org/p/cgr/cgsser/05-02.html.

Fishbein, M. & Ajzen, I. (1975). *Belief, Attitude, Intention, and Behavior.* Reading, MA: Addison-Wesley.

Fishbein, M., Triandis, H.C., Kanfer, F.H., Becker, M., Middlestadt, S.E. & Eichler, A. (2001). Factors influencing behaviour and behaviour change. In A. Baum, T.A. Revenson & J.E. Singer (Eds.), *Handbook of Health Psychology* (pp. 3–17). Mahwah, NJ: Lawrence Erlbaum Associates.

Ford, E.S., Merritt, R.K., Heath, G.W., Powell, K.E., Washburn, R.A., Kriska, A. & Haile, G. (1991). Physical activity behaviors in lower and higher socioeconomic status populations. *American Journal of Epidemiology, 133*(12), 1246–1256.

Fu, F., Rosenbloom, D.I., Wang, L. & Nowak, M.A. (2011). Imitation dynamics of vaccination behaviour on social networks. *Proceedings of the Royal Society of London B: Biological Sciences, 278*(1702), 42–49.

Gallivan, J., Lising, M., Ammary, N.J. & Greenberg, R. (2007). The National Diabetes Education Program's 'Control Your Diabetes. For Life.' campaign: design, implementation, and lessons learned. *Social Marketing Quarterly, 13*, 65–82.

Glider, P., Midyett, S.J., Mills-Novoa, B., Johannessen, K. & Collins, C. (2001). Challenging the collegiate rite of passage: a campus-wide social marketing media campaign to reduce binge drinking. *Journal of Drug Education, 31*(2), 207–220.

Godin, G., Conner, M. & Sheeran, P. (2005). Bridging the intention-behavior 'gap': the role of moral norm. *British Journal of Social Psychology, 44*, 497–512.

Godin, G., Conner, M., Sheeran, P., Bélanger-Gravel, A., Nolin, B. & Gallani, M.C. (2010). Social structure, social cognition, and physical activity: a test of four models. *British Journal of Health Psychology, 15,* 79–95. doi: 10.1348/135910709X429901.

Goodwin, A., Thomas, L., Kirley, B., Hall, W., O'Brien, N. & Hill, K. (2015). *Countermeasures that Work: A Highway Safety Countermeasure Guide for State Highway Safety Offices* (8th edn). Report No. DOT HS 812 202. Washington, DC: National Highway Traffic Safety Administration.

Gordon, R., McDermott, L., Stead, M. & Angus, K. (2006). The effectiveness of social marketing interventions for health improvement: what's the evidence? *Public Health, 120*(12), 1133–1139.

Grant, A.M. & Hofmann, D.A. (2011). It's not all about me: motivating hand hygiene among health care professionals by focusing on patients. *Psychological Science, 22*, 1494–1499.

Grier, S. & Bryant, C. (2005). Social marketing in public health. *Annual Review of Public Health, 26*, 319–339.

Haines, M.P., Barker, G. & Rice, R. (2003). Using social norms to reduce alcohol and tobacco use in two midwestern high schools. In H.W. Perkins (Ed.), *The Social Norms Approach to Preventing School and College Age Substance Abuse: A Handbook for Educators, Counselors, and Clinicians* (pp. 235–244). San Francisco: Jossey-Bass.

Hanks, A. S., Just, D.R., Smith, L.E. & Wansink, B. (2012). Healthy convenience: nudging students toward healthier choices in the lunchroom. *Journal of Public Health, 34*(3), 370–376.

Hardin, G. (1968). The tragedy of the commons. *Science, 162*, 1243–1248.

Highway Loss Data Institute. (2010). Texting laws and collision claim frequencies. *Highway Loss Data Institute Bulletin.* Retrieved on June 30, 2017 from: www.iihs.org/media/fc495300-6f8c-419d-c3b94d178e5a/enPLrA/HLDI%20Research/Bulletins/hldi_bulletin_27.11.pdf.

Hong, S.M. & Page, S. (1989). A psychological reactance scale: development, factor structure and reliability. *Psychological Reports, 64*(3 suppl), 1323–1326.

Johnson, E.J. & Goldstein, D. (2003). Do defaults save lives? *Science, 302*(5649), 1338–1339.

Jung, J.Y. & Mellers, B.A. (2016). American attitudes toward nudges. *Judgment And Decision Making, 11(1)*, 62–74.

Kahneman, D. (2011). *Thinking, Fast and Slow.* New York: Farrar, Straus, and Giroux.

Kenworthy, J.B. & Miller, N. (2001). Perceptual asymmetry in consensus estimates of majority and minority members. *Journal of Personality and Social Psychology, 80*(4), 597–610.

Kikumbih, N., Hanson, K., Mills, A., Mponda, H. & Schellenberg, J.A. (2005). The economics of social marketing: the case of mosquito nets in Tanzania. *Social Science & Medicine*, *60*(2), 369–381.

Kosters, M. & Van der Heijden, J. (2015). From mechanism to virtue: evaluating Nudge theory. *Evaluation: The International Journal of Theory, Research and Practice*, *21*(3), 276–291. doi: 10.1177/1356389015590218.

Krueger, J. & Clement, R.W. (1994). The truly false consensus effect: an ineradicable and egocentric bias in social perception. *Journal of Personality and Social Psychology*, *67*(4), 596–610.

Kubacki, K., Rundle-Thiele, S., Pang, B. & Buyucek, N. (2015). Minimizing alcohol harm: a systematic social marketing review (2000–2014). *Journal of Business Research*, *68*(10), 2214–2222.

Langford, R. & Panter-Brick, C. (2013). A health equity critique of social marketing: where interventions have impact but insufficient reach. *Social Science & Medicine*, *83*, 133–141.

Levy, D.E., Riis, J., Sonnenberg, L.M., Barraclough, S.J. & Thorndike, A.N. (2012). Food choices of minority and low-income employees: a cafeteria intervention. *American Journal of Preventive Medicine*, *43*(3), 240–248. doi: 10.1016/j.amepre.2012.05.004.

Long, T., Taubenheim, A.M., Wayman, J., Temple, S. & Ruoff, B.A. (2008). The heart truth: using the power of branding and social marketing to increase awareness of heart disease in women. *Social Marketing Quarterly*, *14*(3), 3–29.

Luca, N.R. & Suggs, L.S. (2013). Theory and model use in social marketing health interventions. *Journal of Health Communication*, *18*(1), 20–40.

Michie, C. (2016). Childhood obesity: enough discussion, time for action. *British Journal of Diabetes*, *16*(1), 4–5.

Michie, S., Richardson, M., Johnston, M., Abraham, C., Francis, J., Hardeman, W., Eccles, M.P., Cane, J. & Wood, C.E. (2013). The behavior change technique taxonomy (v1) of 93 hierarchically clustered techniques: building an international consensus for the reporting of behavior change interventions. *Annals of Behavioral Medicine*, *46*, 81–95.

Miller, G.F., Gupta, S., Kropp, J.D., Grogan, K.A. & Mathews, A. (2016). The effects of pre-ordering and behavioral nudges on national school lunch program participants' food item selection. *Journal of Economic Psychology*, *55*, 4–16. doi: 10.1016/j.joep.2016.02.010.

Moreira, M.T., Smith, L.A. & Foxcroft, D. (2009). Social norms interventions to reduce alcohol misuse in university or college students. *Cochrane Database of Systematic Reviews*, Issue 3. Art. No.: CD006748. doi: 10.1002/14651858.CD006748.pub2.

Nandi, A., Glymour, M.M. & Subramanian, S.V. (2014). Association among socioeconomic status, health behaviors, and all-cause mortality in the United States. *Epidemiology*, *25*(2), 170–177.

O'Brien, K.M. (2012). Healthy, wealthy, wise? Psychosocial factors influencing the socioeconomic status–health gradient. *Journal of Health Psychology*, *17*(8), 1142–1151.

Peterson, M., Abraham, A. & Waterfield, A. (2005). Marketing physical activity: lessons learned from a statewide media campaign. *Health Promotion Practice*, *6*, 437–446.

Petrescu, D.C., Hollands, G.J., Couturier, D.L., Ng, Y.L. & Marteau, T.M. (2016). Public acceptability in the UK and USA of nudging to reduce obesity: the example of reducing sugar-sweetened beverages consumption. *PLOS ONE*, *11*(6), e0155995.

Prestwich, A., Kellar, I., Conner, M., Lawton, R., Gardner, P. & Turgut, L. (2016). Does changing social influence engender changes in alcohol intake? A meta-analysis. *Journal of Consulting and Clinical Psychology*, *84*, 845–860.

Prochaska, J.O. & DiClemente, C.C. (1986). Toward a comprehensive model of change. In W.R. Miller & N. Heather (Eds.), *Treating Addictive Behaviors* (pp. 3–27). New York: Plenum Press.

Rachlin, H. (2015). Choice architecture: a review of *Why Nudge: The Politics of Libertarian Paternalism*. *Journal of the Experimental Analysis of Behavior*, *104*(2), 198–203. doi: 10.1002/jeab.163.

Richert, M.L., Webb, A.J., Morse, N.A., O'Toole, M.L. & Brownson, C.A. (2007). Move more diabetes: using lay health educators to support physical activity in a community based chronic disease self-management program. *The Diabetes Educator*, *33*(Suppl 16), 179S–184S.

Robinson, E., Benwell, H. & Higgs, S. (2013). Food intake norms increase and decrease snack food intake in a remote confederate stud. *Appetite*, *65*(1), 20–24.

Robinson, E., Thomas, J., Aveyard, P. & Higgs, S. (2014). What everyone else is eating: a systematic review and meta-analysis of the effect of informational eating norms on eating behavior. *Journal of the Academy of Nutrition and Dietetics*, *114*(3), 414–429.

Rutherford, W.H. (1985). The medical effects of seat-belt legislation in the United Kingdom: a critical review of the findings. *Archives of Emergency Medicine*, *2*(4), 221–223.

Scarapicchia, T.M., Sabiston, C.M., Brownrigg, M., Blackburn-Evans, A., Cressy, J., Robb, J. & Faulkner, G.E. (2015). MoveU? Assessing a social marketing campaign to promote physical activity. *Journal of American College Health*, *63*(5), 299–306.

Schwartz, S.H. (1977). Normative influence on altruism. In L. Berkowitz (Ed.), *Advances in Experimental Social Psychology, Vol. 10* (pp. 221–279). New York: Academic Press.

Schwartz, S.H. & Howard, J.A. (1984). Internalized values as moderators of altruism. In E. Staub, D. Bar-Tal, J. Karylowski & J. Reykowski (Eds.), *Development and Maintenance of Prosocial Behavior* (pp. 229–255). New York: Plenum.

Smith, D.V. & Delgado, M.R. (2015). Social nudges: utility conferred from others. *Nature Neuroscience*, *18*(6), 791–792.

Spotswood, F., French, J., Tapp, A. & Stead, M. (2012). Some reasonable but uncomfortable questions about social marketing. *Journal of Social Marketing*, *2*(3), 163–175.

Stasson, M. & Fishbein, M. (1990). The relation between perceived risk and preventive action: a within subject analysis of perceived driving risk and intentions to wear seatbelts. *Journal of Applied Social Psychology*, *20*(19), 1541–1557.

Strack, F. & Deutsch, R. (2004). Reflective and impulsive determinants of social behavior. *Personality and Social Psychology Review*, *8*(3), 220–247.

Stringhini, S., Sabia, S., Shipley, M., Brunner, E., Nabi, H., Kivimaki, M. & Singh-Manoux, A. (2010). Association of socioeconomic position with health behaviors and mortality. *Journal of the American Medical Association*, *303*, 1159–1166.

Sundquist, J., Malmstrom, M. & Johansson, S.E. (1999). Cardiovascular risk factors and the neighbourhood environment: a multilevel analysis. *International Journal of Epidemiology*, *28*, 841–845.

Sunstein, C.R. (2015). Nudges, agency, and abstraction: a reply to critics. *Review of Philosophy and Psychology*, *6*(3), 511–529. doi: 10.1007/s13164-015-0266-z.

Sutton, S.R. & Eiser, J.R. (1990). The decision to wear a seat belt: the role of cognitive factors, fear and prior behaviour. *Psychology and Health*, *4*(2), 111–123.

Thaler, R. & Sunstein, C. (2008). *Nudge: Improving Decisions about Health, Wealth, and Happiness*. London: Penguin.

Thomas, S., Fayter, D., Misso, K., Ogilvie, D., Petticrew, M., Sowden, A., ... & Worthy, G. (2008). Population tobacco control interventions and their effects on social inequalities in smoking: systematic review. *Tobacco Control*, *17*(4), 230–237.

Thorndike, A.N., Riis, J., Sonnenberg, L.M. & Levy, D.E. (2014). Traffic-light labels and choice architecture: promoting healthy food choices. *American Journal of Preventive Medicine*, *46*(2), 143–149. doi: 10.1016/j.amepre.2013.10.002.

Thorndike, A.N., Sonnenberg, L., Riis, J., Barraclough, S. & Levy, D.E. (2012). A 2-phase labeling and choice architecture intervention to improve healthy food and beverage choices. *American Journal of Public Health*, *102*(3), 527–533. doi: 10.2105/AJPH.2011.300391.

VanEpps, E.M. & Roberto, C.A. (2016). The influence of sugar sweetened beverage warnings: a randomized trial of adolescents' choices and beliefs. *American Journal of Preventive Medicine*, *51*(5), 664–672.

Vartanian, L.R., Schwartz, M.B. & Brownell, K.D. (2007). Effects of soft drink consumption on nutrition and health: a systematic review and meta-analysis. *American Journal of Public Health*, *97*(4), 667–675.

Wiltshire, S., Bancroft, A., Amos, A. & Parry, O. (2001). 'They're doing people a service' – qualitative study of smoking, smuggling, and social deprivation. *BMJ*, *323*, 203–207.

Wrigley, N. (2002). 'Food deserts' in British cities: policy context and research priorities. *Urban Studies*, *39*(11), 2029–2040.

6 Self-as-Doer Identity and Health Behavior Change Within Non-Clinical Populations

Adopting and maintaining healthy lifestyle behaviors is key to acquiring optimal health (Loef & Walach, 2012; Nicklett et al., 2012; Riekert, Ockene, & Pbert, 2014; Thorpe et al., 2013). Researchers have identified several health behaviors (e.g., getting regular physical activity, eating a healthy diet, smoking cessation, and limited alcohol consumption) that contribute to better health and the reduction of disease risk (Ford, Zhao, Tsai, & Li, 2011; Riekert et al., 2014). Moreover, researchers have found that engaging in a combination of these health behaviors has the potential to reduce mortality risks by 66% (Loef & Walach, 2012). Although the importance of engaging in a variety of healthy lifestyle behaviors is well documented, few individuals successfully engage in needed health behavior changes and of those that do, sustaining that change proves difficult. For example, those who enroll in weight loss programs are often successful in the short term, but then gain the lost weight back within 3–5 years (Avenell et al., 2004; Dombrowski, Knittle, Avenell, Araujo-Soares, & Sniehotta, 2014; Foster et al., 2010). Smoking cessation programs have similar results with many individuals relapsing within 6 months (Agboola, Mcneill, Coleman, & Leonardi, 2010; Jones, Lewis, Parrot, Wormall, & Coleman, 2016). Physical activity and diet interventions have been found to have some promise with behavior change, but are still limited in the degree to which that change is maintained overtime, especially for physical activity (Fjeldsoe, Neuhaus, Winkler, & Eakin, 2011; Kroeze, Werkman, & Brug, 2006). Given that 40% of premature deaths can be accounted for by suboptimal health behaviors (Spruijt-Metz et al., 2015), finding ways to motivate change and maintenance of that change are vital for achieving good health. As has been argued thus far, the self-as-doer identity is likely to be a useful factor in not only creating behavioral change for healthy lifestyle behaviors but also promoting the maintenance of that change. To better understand the how the self-as-doer influences health behaviors and how it can be used within non-clinical populations, the relevant outcomes from two studies, one on physical activity and one with diet, will be discussed.

Self-as-Doer Identity and Physical Activity Behaviors (The Physical Activity Study)

Being physically active on a regular basis is important for achieving optimal health. Individuals who are regularly active benefit from reduced risk of various diseases, improved mood, and generally enjoy a longer life expectancy (Center for Disease Control, 2015). However, as with many healthy lifestyle behaviors, there are several barriers (e.g., lack of time and motivation, monetary costs, fatigue, lack of social support, etc.) that prevent individuals from making and sustaining the behavior change needed to reduce risk and improve health (Barnidge et al., 2013; Joseph, Ainsworth, Keller, & Dodgson, 2015; Macniven et al., 2014; Martins, Marques, Sarmento, & da Costa, 2015). Likewise, motivation for behavior change may be low and, consequently, individuals lack the needed impetus to continue efforts at behavior change.

Given that a self-as-doer identity provides motivation to engage in behaviors, particularly when they are not reinforcing, Brouwer (n.d.) conducted a cross-sectional study to determine the role that self-as-doer identity has in overcoming barriers for physical activity and how doer identity is related to existing motivational constructs that affect physical activity behaviors. In this study, participants completed questions assessing their motivations for exercise, exercise identity, self-efficacy for exercise behaviors, and self-efficacy for overcoming barriers to exercising. Participants also reviewed educational materials about physical activity behaviors (i.e., the *Physical Activity Guidelines for Americans* published by the Department of Health and Human Services, 2008) and completed the self-as-doer measure (see Chapter 3 in this volume for an overview of this protocol). For the self-as-doer measure, participants were asked to develop six physical activity-specific goals and to then transform those goals into doer identities. Priming participants with the *Physical Activity Guidelines for Americans* was important for their creation of goals and doer identities in that it provided a resource for knowing what good and recommended physical activity behaviors look like. Moreover, it gave many examples of physical activities that could be specified to each individual's current levels of physical activity. Although the introduction of this material may have affected the creation of doer phrases in that many of the phrases corresponded perfectly with the recommendations (see Chapter 3 in this volume for examples of doer identities), the benefits of the educational primer, particularly that participants would have goals that adequately and appropriately reflected the target behavior, outweighed these disadvantages and served to assist participants in creating doer identities that could be used to motivate and sustain the type of physical activity that would lead to health benefits and disease risk reduction. After creating doer identities, participants then rated each doer identity on a 1 ("does not describe me well at all") to 5 ("describes me very well") scale for the degree to which the identity currently described them. Participants created diverse doer identities that described a broad range of physical activity behaviors (e.g., "weight lifter," "runner," "rollerblader") and modifications to their environments to support the changes in those behaviors (e.g., "minimal TV watcher," "taker of the long path," "goal setter"; see Chapter 3 for an in-depth analysis of the created doer identities for physical activity behaviors).

Predicting Physical Activity Behavior

To use doer identification in a way that would be meaningful for helping individuals engage in healthy lifestyle behaviors, is it important that self-as-doer identity can predict corresponding behavioral engagement in ways that existing factors do not. As such, Brouwer (n.d.) ran a hierarchical liner regression to determine whether self-as-doer identity could predict physical activity over and above existing motivational constructs (self-determinism, exercise motivations, exercise identity, and self-efficacy). Self-as-doer identity was a significant predictor, predicting an additional 1.9% of the variance in physical activity behaviors after controlling for the aforementioned constructs, $\Delta R^2 = .019$, $\Delta F\ (1, 197) = 5.77$, $p = .02$.[1] In this way, the self-as-doer can help us to understand why individuals may or may not engage in physical activity behaviors in ways that other constructs cannot.

Overall, findings suggest that doer identification has a unique role in health behavior engagement. Accordingly, researchers and interventionists can use the doer identity in ways that compliment and go beyond existing theories. If the self-as-doer identity can predict physical activity behaviors because, as the self-as-doer theory suggests, doer identification activates a cognitive process which provides motivation for engaging in a behavior, then it likely to be easily transferred to other important healthy lifestyle behaviors (e.g., weight loss, smoking cessation, safe sex practices). For example, if an existing intervention for weight loss is focused on increasing one's self-efficacy, yet the effects of the intervention are not as strong as desired, one might consider also addressing identity associated with doing weight loss behaviors. That is to say, seeing oneself as a "weight loser" or a "healthy weight maintainer" might provide the extra motivation needed to do the behavior and consequently see the desired results.

Relationships Among Doer Identification and Motivational Constructs

In addition to determining whether self-as-doer identity can predict physical activity behaviors beyond existing motivational constructs, the relationship between doer identity and exercise motivations, exercise identity, and self-efficacy for physical activity behaviors was also explored. Knowing how doer identification is related to these constructs can give researchers and interventionists a better picture of how to use it in promoting health behavior change.

Exercise Motivations

The relationship between the self-as-doer identity and motivations to exercise was examined in order to determine whether the self-as-doer identity was a unique motivational construct in predicting physical activity behaviors and how self-as-doer identity was related to various types of exercise motivations. The Exercise Motivations Index-2 (Markland & Ingledew, 1997) measures 14 different reasons for why people engage in physical activity. Doer identification was found to positively and significantly correlate with psychological motives (stress management, revitalization, enjoyment, and exercise as a challenge), social motives (social affiliation, social recognition, and competition needs), and fitness motives (strength, endurance, and nimbleness) for exercise. It was not correlated with body related motives (weight management and appearance) or health motives that emphasized negative outcomes (health pressures and ill-health avoidance). It was, however, positively correlated with the "positive health" health motive. Correlation coefficients can be found in Table 4.1.

Although most of the correlations were similar in strength (i.e., .18–.33), doer identity most strongly correlated with the challenge and affiliation motives. First, self-as-doer identity was specifically related to motivations

Table 4.1 Correlations between self-as-doer identity and exercise motivations

	Exercise motivations													
	Stress	*Revitalization*	*Enjoyment*	*Challenge*	*Social-recognition*	*Affiliation*	*Competition*	*Health pressures*	*Ill-health avoidance*	*Positive health*	*Weight management*	*Appearance*	*Strength and endurance*	*Nimbleness*
Self-as-doer	.21**	.21**	.26***	.33***	.22***	.30***	.23***	.06	.12	.17*	–.05	.06	.27***	.18**

* p <.05;
**p <.01;
*** p < .001.

that focus on physical activity as a means of having a personal challenge to face or developing personal skills and exploring limits of one's body. These motivations are clearly in line with the self-as-doer theory in that doer identity is focused on behavior based upon goals that promote personal betterment. Second, the self-as-doer was related to affiliation motives, which corresponds to wanting to include others in physical activities. For instance, individuals exercise to spend time with friends, to have fun being active with other people, and to make new friends. Although it is argued that the self-as-doer is primarily focused on the self, it may be that doer identification is strengthened by sharing that identity with others or that by participating in physical activity with others, one begins to take cues from the social environment and modify their self-concept as the doer of their behaviors accordingly. Overall, if one were to develop an intervention for physical activity, it would be valuable to consider how doer identity might promote these forms of motivations or that individuals with such motivations might be more likely to develop doer identities related to physical activity.

As it relates to motivations for physical activity behaviors, the self-as-doer is theoretically supported in that it is associated with diverse motives (i.e., psychology, social, and fitness) that involve more self-determined behaviors (e.g., enjoyment, challenge, skill improvement, affiliation, positive health etc.). That the self-as-doer was not associated with motivations that emphasize negative outcomes like ill-health avoidance or external motivations like health pressures further supports the notion that doer identity is focused on internal motivation for actively engaging in physical behavior. Additionally, the lack of relationships with appearance and weight maintenance might suggest that doer identity is associated with linking the self with the behavior and not just the self-concept. Both appearance and weight maintenance motivations are primarily reflective of the image of the self (e.g., "look more attractive," "have a good body," to stay slim") rather than a performing a behavior. In sum, the self-as-doer identity is related to diverse exercise motivations that align with more self-determined behaviors, but is arguably a distinct form of motivation for physical activity behaviors.

Exercise Identity

Exercise-specific identity has been associated with greater frequency of physical activity behaviors (Grant, Hogg, & Crano, 2015; Miller, Ogletree, & Welshimer, 2002; Reifsteck, Gill, & Labban, 2016; Strachan, Brawley, Spink, & Jung, 2009; Wilson & Muon, 2008). Exercise identity, as conceptualized by Anderson and Cychosz (1994) in their Exercise Identity Scale and later modified by Wilson and Muon (2008), is comprised of identity roles (e.g., "Others see me as someone who exercises regularly") and exercise beliefs (e.g., “I have numerous goals related to exercising”). Although theoretically similar, the self-as-doer is different in that it represents the active agent of the behavior, not just the roles one might have or the beliefs one might hold about exercise behaviors. What makes the self-as-doer unique is the connecting of one’s self-concept with the physical activity behavior. To assess the degree of overlap between exercise identity and a self-as-doer identity, the self-as-doer was correlated with exercise identity (Brouwer, n.d.). Results demonstrated that the self-as-doer identity was positively and significantly correlated with the role identity (.39, $p < .001$) and exercise beliefs ($r = .29, p < .001$) subscales of the Exercise Identity Scale. That doer identification was positively correlated with both subscales suggests that doer identification is associated with both exercise roles and beliefs. That is, a stronger doer identity is related to a stronger likelihood of endorsing exercise roles and participatory beliefs about exercise. However, that the correlation was only a medium effect supports the idea that the self-as-doer is not the same construct as exercise roles and beliefs.

Self-Efficacy

Self-efficacy, the belief in one’s ability to perform a behavior, plays a vital role in predicting health behaviors (Bandura, 1998; Luszczynska et al., 2016; Nezami et al., 2016; Sheeran et al., 2016), especially physical activity behaviors (Olander et al., 2013; Higgins, Middleton, Winner, & Janelle, 2014; Shieh, Weaver, Hanna, Newsome, & Mogos, 2015). To ascertain the relationship between self-as-doer identity and self-efficacy for general physical activity and self-efficacy for overcoming barriers related to physical activity, correlations were computed. Results demonstrated that stronger doer identification was associated with greater self-efficacy for engaging in physical activity behaviors ($r = .17, p = .01$) and for overcoming barriers to physical activity behaviors ($r = .25, p < .001$). In general, results demonstrate that doer identity is positively associated with the degree of confidence one feels about their abilities to engage in physical activity and to overcome barriers associated with physical activity. Again, results affirm the self-as-doer theory in that the self-as-doer identity is positively related to other factors which have a predictive relationship with physical activity behaviors.

In sum, the self-as-doer identity can predict physical activity above and beyond other motivational constructs and is associated with exercise identity roles and beliefs, and self-efficacy for both physical activity behaviors in general and for overcoming barriers. The generally positive and moderate relationships that self-as-doer identity has with exercise identity, self-efficacy, and motivations for exercise suggests that self-as-doer identity is a distinct factor that can be used alongside of these constructs without being superfluous and therefore strengthening the ability to determine what contributes to health behavior change and maintenance. Although our conclusions about these relationships are specific to physical activity behaviors, the nature and theory of the self-as-doer identity suggests that such findings can be generalized to other healthy lifestyle behaviors (e.g., weight loss, safe sex practices, smoking cessation, etc.)

It is important to note, however, that this work is limited in that it is correlational and it is not possible to determine whether engaging in physical activity increases one's identification with a behavior or whether the development of an identity as the doer of one's behavior causes behavior change. In an effort to determine whether manipulating the self-as-doer identity could lead to corresponding behavior change, Brouwer and Mosack (2015) developed an intervention aimed at activating self-as-doer identities and tested whether it would cause a change in diet behaviors and whether this behavior change could be maintained.

Self-as-Doer Identity and Diet Behaviors (The Healthy Eating Study)

The self-as-doer intervention was developed from the idea that conceptualizing the degree to which one identifies with goals and behavior related to certain behavior change (e.g., more fruit consumption) and discussing the discrepancies between one's current identification (i.e., a poor fruit eater) and what it might take to define oneself to a stronger degree in relation to the behavior in question (e.g., purchase more fruits to become a better fruit eater) could be a means to bring about change in behavioral intention and behavior (O'Keefe, 2002). The processes whereby individuals identify goals related to healthy eating and transform those goals into identity statements (i.e., the self-as-doer) was projected to have the potential to activate existing self-representations related to healthy eating. Furthermore, the cognitive process of conceptualizing what it means to be a "healthy eater" can bring about greater identification with different, more health consistent behaviors which may consequently promote behavior change. Therefore, the primary objectives of the self-as-doer intervention were to assist participants with developing goals related to healthy eating behaviors, transforming those goals into self-as-doer identity statements, and then reflecting on the degree to which doer identities were descriptive of oneself.

For the experimental evaluation of the intervention, participants were asked to complete the self-as-doer measure and then answer a few questions related to the doer identities they created (Brouwer & Mosack, 2015). As was described in the physical activity study, prior to competing the self-as-doer measure, participants reviewed educational information. For this study, however, it was nutritional education in the form of pamphlets and brochures created by the United States Department of Agriculture (USDA, 2010a, 2010b, 2010c). As before, the educational material served as both a prime and a resource to assist participants in generating appropriate goals; however, for this study, the goals were specific to healthy eating behaviors. Although the focus of the study was to measure the degree of change in fruit, vegetable, whole grain, low-fat dairy, and sugar-sweetened beverage consumption, participants were not restricted in the types of healthy eating goals that they could create (see Chapter 3 for details on created doer phrases). The methods for creating doer identities and rating those doer identities in terms of how well each created identity described the participant were similar to that described previously in the physical activity study.

Upon completion of the self-as-doer measure, the interviewer then began the process of helping the participant reflect on the degree to which doer identities were consistent with their current self-concept and, if not, how one would go about enhancing that consistency. For this process (and as has been described previously in Brouwer & Mosack, 2015), the interviewer selected one of the created doer identities and asked participants to envision themselves as the doer of the "-er" phrase they constructed. For example, the researcher might say, "Picture yourself being a fruit eater. What would that look like?" Participants were then allowed time to verbally describe the form that this doer identity took for them. After this description, the researcher then identified how the participant rated that particular identity and asked them how they could see themselves as that doer identity to a greater degree in subsequent weeks. For example, the interviewer would say, "I see that you rated yourself as a 'fruit eater' as a 2 (does not describe me well). What would it take in this next week and beyond this next week to see yourself as a fruit eater to a greater degree, say a 4 or a 5 instead of a 2?" This process was repeated for 3 or 4 of the created doer identities. Participants were then provided with a verbal summary of the task and encouraged to think about their doer identities as they made diet choices in later weeks (Brouwer & Mosack, 2015).

The outcomes of the study were measured by having participants complete food diaries 1 week before the intervention, 1 week after the intervention and then again 1 month following the intervention. The study lasted approximately 6 weeks and a healthy diet was operationalized as increases in one's consumption of fruits, vegetables, whole grains, and low-fat dairy and a reduction in sugar-sweetened beverage consumption. The diets of those who received the self-as-doer intervention were compared to a nutrition education group (i.e., those who read the aforementioned USDA nutrition education pamphlets) and a control group (i.e., those who received no intervention; see Brouwer & Mosack, 2015 for a detailed description of the study hypotheses and procedures).

Dietary Change Results

Results demonstrated that the self-as-doer intervention was an effective tool to promote maintenance of overall healthy eating behaviors. Participants who completed the intervention had significantly[2] higher rates of overall healthy food consumption at the one-month follow-up than did those who received only nutrition education ((t[116]= 2.19, p = .09) and those in the control group (t[116] = 2.53, p = .04). The effect of the intervention for specific food groups was mixed. There were no specific effects for fruit and vegetable consumption, but there were some significant changes across time and significant differences between groups for whole grain, low-fat dairy, and sugar-sweetened beverage consumption (see Figure 4.1).

Participants who completed the self-as-doer intervention significantly increased their whole grain consumption from baseline to post-intervention.

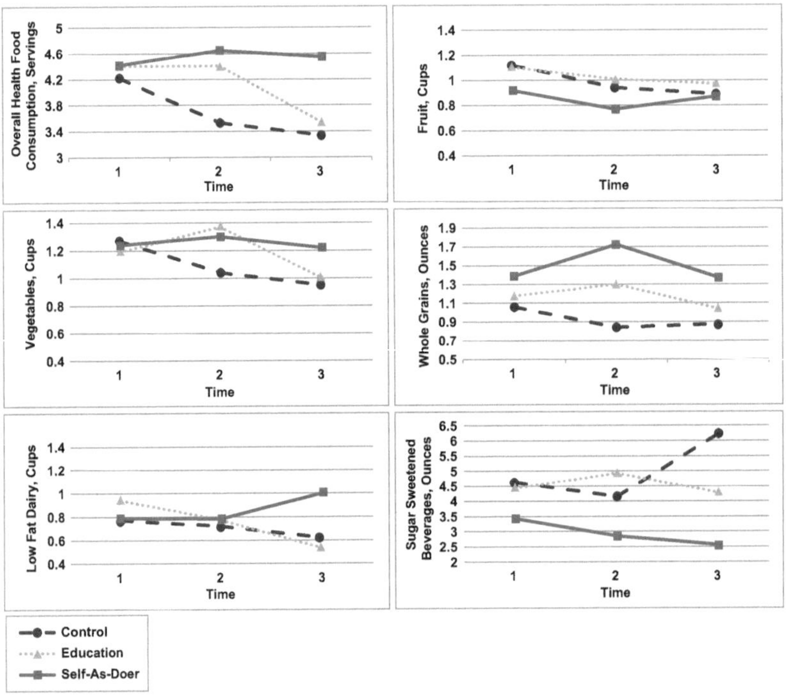

Figure 4.1 Change across time and differences among groups for overall and food-group specific health food consumption

Source: From "Motivating health diet behaviors: The self-as-doer identity" by A. M. Brouwer and K. E. Mosack, 2015, *Self and Identity, 14*, p. 648.Copyright [2015] by Taylor & Francis. Reprinted with permission.

This increase, coinciding with a significant decrease in whole grain consumption in the control group, led to a significant difference between those who had the self-as-doer intervention and those in the control group one week after the intervention, $t(116)= 3.40$, $p = 003$. There was, however, a significant decrease in whole grain consumption for the self-as-doer intervention group, returning their consumption back to baseline rates at the one-month follow-up time period. For low-fat dairy consumption, participants who received the intervention had significant increases in their consumption rates between the week after the intervention and the one-month follow-up, $t[116] = 2.26$, $p = .08$. At one-month follow-up, those who received the self-as-doer intervention had significantly higher low-fat dairy consumption than those who received nutrition education ($t[116] = 2.62$, $p = .03$) and lower sugar-sweetened beverage consumption than did those in the control group, $t(116) = 2.63$, $p = .03$.

Overall, the findings demonstrated that although the self-as-doer intervention did not increase healthy food consumption, it did cause participants to maintain a higher level of healthy eating behaviors compared to those who only received nutrition education and those who received no intervention (Brouwer & Mosack, 2015). As such, using the self-as-doer intervention could play and important role in promoting the maintenance of other healthy lifestyle behaviors. For example, perhaps an individual is considering losing weight or maintaining weight loss but has struggled to do so. It may be that adopting an identity as a "weight loser" or a "healthy weight maintainer" and then reflecting on how one could see oneself as that identity to a stronger degree could create the added motivation needed to not just change but also maintain these health behaviors. The same could be said for smoking behaviors. If an individual wants to quit smoking, but is facing barriers in being able to maintain a reduction in smoking, developing goals and corresponding self-as-doer identities to reduce and eventually quit smoking (e.g., "smoking reducer," "one cigarette a day smoker," "smoking quitter") could provide the added motivation to overcome the barriers that initially prevented the behavior change and that caused relapse in the unwanted behavior.

The self-as-doer intervention caused participants to maintain their overall healthy eating behaviors but had less consistent effects for specific food groups. Participants may have focused on changing one or two diet behaviors at a time, making finding statistical significance for all diet behaviors difficult (Brouwer & Mosack, 2015). As a result, further interventions might focus more specifically on addressing certain foods rather than on the broader behavior of eating a healthy diet. The specificity might help individuals focus on a single identity that can be translated more successfully into behavior change. Participants may have also had insufficient knowledge about nutrition to increase their healthy food consumption in a statistically measurable degree. One participant, for example, chose to make dietary changes related to fruit and whole grain consumption by drinking more fruit juice and eating certain granola bars because the packaging advertised that they were made from whole grains. Unfortunately the juice she chose contained only 10% fruit juice and the amount of whole grains in each granola bar was very small, only 0.25 ounces. As such, her behavior changed, but not in a sufficiently measurable form (Brouwer & Mosack, 2015). One could argue that for cases such as these, the self-as-doer intervention did have a meaningful change in health behavior. Going forward with the intervention, it may be important to provide adequate and accurate nutritional information so that participants are clear on what constitutes a measurable change in each of their behavioral goals and what pitfalls are common when making healthy food decisions (e.g., false advertising). For example, one could provide a list of foods which have the highest whole grain amounts or vegetables that are considered to be more highly nutritious than others (e.g., dark green and orange vegetables vs. lettuce).

Results of the Intervention Impact

Participants' responses, both solicited and unsolicited, to the self-as-doer intervention were also recorded in an effort to better understand the most salient parts of the self-as-doer intervention (Brouwer & Mosack, 2015). First, participants reported adopting their doer identities and using them to make healthy diet choices. In an unsolicited email one participant described how she was "excited to become a 'leafy vegetable eater'," a doer-identity phrase she created at the time of the self-as-doer intervention. Another participant, without prompting, wrote the created doer identities next to foods that supported that identity in her food diaries. For example, she wrote "veggie grabber" next to foods such as celery and carrots that she ate. Another participant who saw herself as a "quinoa eater" also found that part of that identity includes sharing her recipe discoveries with others. After the lab visit where she created doer identities, she brought in a sample of quinoa and tips on how best to serve it as part of one's meal.

Participants also reported how thinking about doer identities helped them to make healthier diet choices. For example, one participant described how she was at a vending machine preparing to get her usual sugar-sweetened beverage, but before making the selection, she thought to herself, "no, I'm a 'less sugar drinker' (a doer identity she had created in the intervention) and should chose a diet beverage instead." The identity as a "less sugar drinker" led her to then choose a diet drink rather than her habitual choice of a sugar-sweetened drink. Defining oneself according to a doer identity also led participants to make healthy choices, even when it was not the preferred choice. For example, at a follow-up visit, one participant inquired about the amount of vegetables in a vegetarian burger. Upon finding out that there was only about one-quarter cup servings of vegetables in the burger she said, "You mean I choked down that veggie burger instead of a hot dog for only a quarter cup of veggies?" (Brouwer & Mosack, 2015).

Overall, the self-as-doer intervention was effective in getting individuals to think about themselves as the doer of their behaviors and from both qualitative and quantitative results, the intervention demonstrates how a motivational identity can promote the maintenance of healthy eating behaviors. Although not all food-group specific healthy eating behaviors were changed over the course of the study, the findings support previous research (Brouwer & Mosack, 2012; Houser-Marko & Sheldon, 2006; RiseSheeran, & Hukkelberg, 2010; Stryker & Burke, 2000) and demonstrate how the self-as-doer identity can be activated through a simple environmental intervention to consequently influence health behavior change and maintenance related to healthy eating.

Conclusion

In this chapter the utility of the self-as-doer in healthy, non-clinical populations has been discussed. Health behavior change and maintenance are difficult, but the self-as-doer provides a motivational identity that can be used to overcome barriers to promote sustaining health behavior enactment. The use of the self-as-doer identity within the context of physical activity behaviors and diet demonstrates that, indeed, a doer identification can predict health behaviors and even promote the maintenance of that behavior. That the self-as-doer is about processing how one sees oneself as the doer of his or her goals gives it universal applicability. The steps of creating goals, transforming those goals into doer statements, and then reflecting on the degree to which on could see oneself as that doer to a stronger degree can be applied to most any healthy lifestyle behavior. The research reviewed in this chapter supports the self-as-doer theory that linking a self-concept to a behavior in order to conceptualize oneself as the doer of one's behavior can have an effect on health behavior, especially maintenance of that behavior. Therefore, there is promise in using the self-as-doer in diverse health behaviors among non-clinical populations. Given its widespread applicability, the self-as-doer could be used, for example, to promote safer sex practices, better sleep habits, participating in disease-prevention screenings, and managing stress in healthy populations. This approach can also be useful to promote improve health behaviors and manage chronic conditions within clinical populations too. To that end, I now turn to discussing how the self-as-doer identity can be used as a disease management tool.

Notes

1. Additional statistical details are available from the author.
2. Bonferroni corrections were performed for all follow-up analyses to control for type I errors. Given that the original study was designed as a pilot study, significance criteria were set at $p = .10$.

References

Agboola, S., Mcneill, A., Coleman, T., & Leonardi, B. J. (2010). A systematic review of the effectiveness of smoking relapse prevention interventions for abstinent smokers. *Addiction, 105*, 1362–1380. doi: 10.1111/j.1360–0443.2010.02996.x

Anderson, D. F., & Cychosz, C. M. (1994). Development of an exercise identity scale. *Perceptual and Motor Skills, 78*(3, Pt 1), 747–751. doi: 10.2466/pms.1994.78.3.747

Avenell, A., Broom, J., Brown, T. J., Poobalan, A., Aucott, L., Stearns, S. C., . . . Grant, A. M. (2004). Systematic review of the long-term effects and economic consequences of treatments for obesity and implications for health improvement. *Health Technology Assessment, 8*(21), 1–182.

Bandura, A. (1998). Health promotion from the perspective of social cognitive theory. *Psychology and Health, 13*, 623–649. doi: 10.1080/08870449808407422

Barnidge, E. K., Radvanyi, C., Duggan, K., Motton, F., Wiggs, I., Baker, E. A., & Brownson, R. C. (2013). Understanding and addressing barriers to implementation of environmental and policy interventions to support physical activity and healthy eating in rural communities. *Journal of Rural Health, 29*(1), 97–105. doi: 10.1111/j.1748–0361.2012.00431.x

Brouwer, A. M. (n.d.). *Predicting physical activity with identity: The self-as-doer identity*. Unpublished manuscript.

Brouwer, A. M., & Mosack, K. E. (2015). Motivating health diet behaviors: The self-as-doer identity. *Self and Identity, 14*, 638–653. doi: 10.1080/15298868.2015.1043335

Center for Disease Control (2015). *The benefits of physical activity*. Retrieved from www.cdc.gov/physicalactivity/basics/pa-health/

Department of Health and Human Services (2008). *2008 physical activity guidelines for Americans*. Retrieved from https://health.gov/paguidelines/pdf/paguide.pdf

Dombrowski, S. U., Knittle, K., Avenell, A., Araujo-Soares, V., & Sniehotta, F. F. (2014). Long-term maintenance of weight loss in obese adults: A systematic review of randomised controlled trials of nonsurgical weight loss maintenance interventions with meta-analyses. *British Medical Journal, 348*, g2646. doi: 10.1136/bmj.g2646

Fjeldsoe, B., Neuhaus, M., Winkler, E., & Eakin, E. (2011). Systematic review of maintenance of behavior change following physical activity and dietary interventions. *Health Psychology, 30*(1), 99–109. doi: 10.1037/a0021974

Ford, E. S., Zhao, G., Tsai, J., & Li, C. (2011). Low-risk lifestyle behaviors and all-cause mortality: Findings from the National Health and Nutrition Examination Survey III Mortality Study. *American Journal of Public Health, 101*(10), 1922–1929. doi: 10.2105/AJPH.2011.300167

Foster, G. D., Wyatt, H. R., Hill, J. O., Makris, A. P., Rosenbaum, D. L., Brill, C., . . . Klein, S. (2010). Weight and metabolic outcomes after 2 years on a low-carbohydrate versus low-fat diet: A randomized trial. *Annals of Internal Medicine, 153*, 147–157. doi: 10.7326/0003-4819-153-3-201008030-00005

Grant, F., Hogg, M. A., & Crano, W. D. (2015). Yes, we can: Physical activity and group identification among healthy adults. *Journal of Applied Social Psychology, 45*(7), 383–390. doi: 10.1111/jasp.12305

Higgins, T. J., Middleton, K. R., Winner, L., & Janelle, C. M. (2014). Physical activity interventions differentially affect exercise task and barrier self-efficacy: A meta-analysis. *Health Psychology, 33*(8), 891–903. doi: 10.1037/a0033864

Houser-Marko, L., & Sheldon, K. M. (2006). Motivating behavioral persistence: The self-as-doer construct. *Personality and Social Psychology Bulletin, 32*, 1037–1049. doi: 10.1177/0146167206287974

Jones, M., Lewis, S., Parrott, S., Wormall, S., & Coleman, T. (2016). Re-starting smoking in the postpartum period after receiving a smoking cessation intervention: A systematic review. *Addiction, 111*(6), 981–990. doi: 10.1111/add.13309

Joseph, R. P., Ainsworth, B. E., Keller, C., & Dodgson, J. E. (2015). Barriers to physical activity among African American women: An integrative review of the literature. *Women & Health, 55*(6), 679–699. doi: 10.1080/03630242.2015.1039184

Kroeze, W., Werkman, A., & Brug, J. (2006). A systematic review of randomized trials on the effectiveness of computer-tailored education on physical activity and dietary behaviors. *Annals of Behavioral Medicine, 31*, 205–223. doi: 10.1207/s15324796abm3103_2

Loef, M., & Walach, H. (2012). The combined effects of healthy lifestyle behaviors on all cause mortality: A systematic review and meta-analysis. *Preventive Medicine: An International Journal Devoted to Practice and Theory, 55*(3), 163–170. doi: 10.1016/j.ypmed.2012.06.017

Luszczynska, A., Horodyska, K., Zarychta, K., Liszewska, N., Knoll, N., & Scholz, U. (2016). Planning and self-efficacy interventions encouraging replacing energy-dense foods intake with fruit and vegetable: A longitudinal experimental study. *Psychology & Health, 31*(1), 40–64. doi: 10.1080/08870446.2015.1070156

Macniven, R., Pye, V., Merom, D., Milat, A., Monger, C., Bauman, A., & van der Ploeg, H. (2014). Barriers and enablers to physical activity among older Australians who want to increase their physical activity levels. *Journal of Physical Activity & Health, 11*(7), 1420–1429. doi: 10.1123/jpah.2012–0096

Markland, D., & Ingledew, D. K. (1997). The measurement of exercise motives: Factorial validity and invariance across gender of a revised exercise motivations inventory. *British Journal of Health Psychology, 2*, 361–376. doi: 10.1111/j.2044 8287.1997.tb00549.x

Martins, J., Marques, A., Sarmento, H., & da Costa, F. C. (2015). Adolescents' perspectives on the barriers and facilitators of physical activity: A systematic review of qualitative studies. *Health Education Research, 30*(5), 742–755. doi: 10.1093/her/cyv042

Miller, K. M., Ogletree, R. J., & Welshimer, K. (2002). Impact of activity behaviors in physical activity identity and self-efficacy. *American Journal of Health Behavior*, *26*, 323–330. doi: 10.5993/AJHB.26.5.1

Nezami, B. T., Lang, W., Jakicic, J. M., Davis, K. K., Polzien, K., Rickman, A. D., . . . Tate, D. F. (2016). The effect of self-efficacy on behavior and weight in a behavioral weight-loss intervention. *Health Psychology*, *35*(7), 714–722. doi: 10.1037/hea0000378

Nicklett, E. J., Semba, R. D., Xue, Q., Tian, J., Sun, K., Cappola, A. R., . . . Fried, L. P. (2012). Fruit and vegetable intake, physical activity, and mortality in older community-dwelling women. *Journal of the American Geriatrics Society*, *60*(5), 862–868. doi: 10.1111/j.1532–5415.2012.03924.x

O'Keefe, D. J. (2002). *Persuasion: Theory and research*. Beverly Hills, CA: Sage.

Olander, E. K., Fletcher, H., Williams, S., Lou, A., Turner, A., & French, D. P. (2013). What are the most effective techniques in changing obese individuals' physical activity self-efficacy and behaviour: A systematic review and meta-analysis. *International Journal of Behavioral Nutrition and Physical Activity*, *10*. doi: 10.1186/1479-5868-10-29

Reifsteck, E. J., Gill, D. L., & Labban, J. D. (2016). "Athletes" and "exercisers": Understanding identity, motivation, and physical activity participation in former college athletes. *Sport, Exercise, and Performance Psychology*, *5*(1), 25–38. doi: 10.1037/spy0000046

Riekert, K. A., Ockene, J. K., & Pbert, L. (Eds.). (2014). *The handbook of health behavior change*. New York: Springer Publishing.

Rise, J., Sheeran, P., & Hukkelberg, S. (2010). The role of self-identity in the theory of planned behavior: A meta-analysis. *Journal of Applied Social Psychology*, *40*, 1085–1105. doi: 10.1111/j.1559–1816.2010.00611.x/pdf

Sheeran, P., Maki, A., Montanaro, E., Avishai-Yitshak, A., Bryan, A., Klein, W. P., . . . Rothman, A. J. (2016). The impact of changing attitudes, norms, and self-efficacy on health-related intentions and behavior: A meta-analysis. *Health Psychology*, *35*(11), 1178–1188. doi: 10.1037/hea0000387

Shieh, C., Weaver, M. T., Hanna, K. M., Newsome, K., & Mogos, M. (2015). Association of self-efficacy and self-regulation with nutrition and exercise behaviors in a community sample of adults. *Journal of Community Health Nursing*, *32*(4), 199–211. doi: 10.1080/07370016.2015.1087262

Spruijt-Metz, D., Hekler, E., Saranummi, N., Intille, S., Korhonen, I., Nilsen, W., . . . Pavel, M. (2015). Building new computational models to support health behavior change and maintenance: New opportunities in behavioral research. *Translational Behavioral Medicine*, *5*(3), 335–346. doi: 10.1007/s13142-015-0324-1

Strachan, S. M., Brawley, L. R., Spink, K. S., & Jung, M. E. (2009). Strength of exercise identity and identity-exercise consistency. *Journal of Health Psychology*, *14*, 1196–1206. doi: 10.1177/1359105309346340

Stryker, S., & Burke, P. J. (2000). The past, present, and future of identity theory. *Social Psychology Quarterly*, *63*, 284–297. Retrieved from www.jstor.org/stable/2695840

Thorpe, R. J., Wilson-Frederick, S. M., Bowie, J. V., Coa, K., Clay, O. J., LaVeist, T. A., & Whitfield, K. E. (2013). Health behaviors and all-cause mortality in African

American men. *American Journal of Men's Health, 7*(4, Suppl.), 8S–18S. doi: 10.1177/1557988313487552

U.S. Department of Agriculture (2010a). *Let's eat for the health of it.* Retrieved from www.choosemyplate.gov/sites/default/files/audiences/DG2010Brochure.pdf

U.S. Department of Agriculture (2010b). *Build a healthy meal.* Retrieved from www.choosemyplate.gov/sites/default/files/tentips/DGTipsheet38BuildHealthyMealtimeHabits_0.pdf

U.S. Department of Agriculture (2010c). *Choose MyPlate 10 tips to a great plate.* Retrieved from www.choosemyplate.gov/sites/default/files/tentips/DGTipsheet1ChooseMyPlate.pdf

Wilson, P. M., & Muon, S. (2008). Psychometric properties of the exercise identity scale in a university sample. *International Journal of Sport and Exercise Psychology, 6*(2), 115–131. doi: 10.1080/1612197X.2008.96718

7

TRUST AND HEALTH

The road to wellness?

This chapter was first published in *The Psychology of Trust* and cross-referencing relates to chapters in the original volume. Please visit www.routledge.com/9781138678491 for more information about the book

The experience of entering an operating theatre highlights the extent to which trust plays a role in medical treatment. Here you are – helpless in the hands of physicians and technology. Humans are increasingly under the care of medical professionals because of advances in medical science and as a result live longer. As in many facets of peoples' lives (see Chapter 1) though, controversies regarding trust in health professionals has emerged in contemporary society.

READ ALL ABOUT IT!

A scientific magazine headline has declared that "America's Trust in Doctors Is Failing" (Harding, 2014, n.p.). The magazine headline was based, in large part, on the paper the by Blendon, Benson, Joachim and Hero (2014). These authors reviewed historical polling data on the public's trust in US physicians and medical leaders from 1966 through 2014. The authors also considered the findings from a 29-country survey conducted from March 2011 through April 2013 as part of the International Social Survey Programme (ISSP). According to their report, the public's trust in the leaders of the US medical profession declined sharply over the past half century, with around 75% of Americans in 1966 saying that they had great confidence in the leaders of the medical profession but only 34% saying so in 2012. According to the paper, public confidence in the US health care system was currently low and only 23% expressed a great deal or quite a lot of confidence in the system. Nevertheless, the report stated the public's current trust in physicians' integrity was high, with 69% of the public rating the honesty and ethical standards of physicians as a group as "very high" or "high". In that vein, around 60% of US adults agreed in the surveys that currently, "All things considered, doctors in [your country] can be trusted" (p. 1570), although adults in some other countries agreed more with the statement. Adults in the US were very satisfied with the quality of the health care they received and ranked third of the countries in patient satisfaction. The authors proposed that the mixed pattern of findings regarding trust was due, in part, to the lack of a universal health care system in the United States.

Is America's trust in doctors failing as the above magazine title states? In my view, no! It is important to highlight, here, the problems with believing headlines. In order to get a more accurate view it is important to read the primary sources – read them very carefully. Nevertheless, the magazine article and primary source attests to the following two problems.

First, they demonstrate the confusion regarding what is a proper measure of trust in physicians/doctors. The magazine article (Harding, 2014) and the publication by Blendon et al. (2014) include an array of different terms such as "trust", "confidence", and "integrity". Although we have an intuitive understanding of these, what did they mean to the respondents and do they assess the same thing? The answer from my perspective is that their meaning is uncertain and the terms are not synonymous. Certainly patient satisfaction is separate from trust in physicians.

Second, the papers highlight the misguided strategy of confusing trust in physicians with trust in the medical system and trust in leaders in the field of medicine. Medical treatment is a multilevel construct with complex links between the leaders in the field of medicine; medical systems (e.g., socialised vs non-socialised); hospitals; treatment centres; consultants, physicians, and nurses in treatment centres; and personal physicians (see Pilgrim, Tomasini, & Vassilev, 2010). The role of trust in medical treatment is indeed complex! This chapter will focus on trust in physicians/doctors and nurses because of its prevalence in psychological research, although there is a broader domain of medical trust (e.g., leaders, systems, etc.) that is important in its own right.

DOES BEING TRUST IN GENERALISED OTHERS INCREASE OUR HEALTH?

Research has shown that the individuals who hold low generalised trust in others (see Generalised Trust Beliefs in Chapter 1) tend have shorter lives. In the study by Barefoot et al. (1998) 100 adults (44 to 80 years of age) were administered measures of generalised trust beliefs (Rotter's GTB scale), psychological well-being, life satisfaction, and functional health (self-rated health and daily activities). Mortality was assessed 14 years later. The researchers found that low generalised trust beliefs were associated with poor psychological adjustment (notably negative emotions); poor functional health, both concurrently and prospectively; and earlier mortality, which tended to be evident even when functional health was statistically controlled. The authors suggested that low generalised trust beliefs were linked to poor health/lower mortality because those relations were the results of such factors as lack of social support, cynicism, reductions in the body's immunity to illness, and unwillingness to seek out needed medical treatment. Nummela, Raivio, and Uutela (2012) have found similar relations in Southern Finland, but only for men.

DOES ADULTS' TRUST IN HEALTH PROFESSIONALS PROMOTE HEALTH?

A number of studies show that adults' trust beliefs in physicians are associated with successful medical treatment. For example, Thom and his colleagues (Thom, Kravitz, Bell, Krupat, & Azari, 2002; Thom, Ribisl, Stewart, Luke, & The Stanford Trust Study Physicians, 1999) found that adults' scores on the Trust in Physicians Scale (TPS) were associated with self-reported continuity with physician, adherence to medication, satisfaction with physician, satisfaction with their care, the intention to follow the doctor's advice, and symptom improvement after two weeks. Similar relations between adults' trust and some health-related measures have been found in studies employing other scales to assess adults' trust beliefs in physicians (see Birkhäuer et al., 2017).

Scholars have been concerned with racial differences in medical treatment as they bear on trust. In particular, researchers have found racial disparities in the treatment of HIV (see Saha, Jacobs, Moore, & Beach, 2010). Black people are less likely to receive antiretroviral therapy (ART) than Caucasian people. Saha et al. (2010) proposed that lower trust in physicians by Black people than Caucasian people would account for their lower medical treatment of AIDS. In the study, 1,327 patients (1,104 Black) rated: (a) how much they trusted their physicians, (b) the quality of their life, (c) quality of patient-provider interaction, and (d) whether they had received ART (cross-checked with clinical records). Also, the patients' CD4 lymphocyte counts were obtained from clinical records. The researchers found that, compared to Caucasian people, Black people were less trusting in their physicians, less likely to receive ART, less likely to adhere to ART, and less likely to achieve viral suppression. Also it was found that trust in physicians was associated with adherence to ART. The findings showed that the Black people who had complete trust in their physicians were similar to Caucasian people in adhering to ART. The researchers argued that racial disparity between Black and Caucasian people in the treatment of HIV is a product, in part, of Black people's low trust in physicians and resulting lack of adherence to ART.

DOES CHILDREN'S/ADOLESCENT'S TRUST IN HEALTH PROFESSIONALS PROMOTE HEALTH?

One answer to this question is provided by the research that my colleagues and I have carried out on children's/adolescents' trust in physicians and nurses. Guided by the BDT Framework, we carried out studies on children (around 10 years of age) to develop a Children's Trust in General Physicians Scale (CTGPS; Rotenberg et al., 2008) and Children's Trust General Nurses Scale (CTGNS; Rotenberg, Woods, & Betts, 2015). The analyses confirmed that the CTGPS and CTGNS assessed the three bases of trust: reliability, emotional, and honesty. As expected, it was found that the CTGPS (notably emotional trust subscale) scores were associated with the reports of how much children trusted doctors, and the children's adherence to prescribed medical regimes. The latter finding yielded support for the principle that trust in physicians promotes adherence. It was found that the CTGNS scores were associated with children's "trust" in, but not "fear" of, nurses. Finally, it was found that the CTGNS were associated with parent's reports of the frequency with which they and their children visited medical centres. The latter finding supported the hypothesis that the more frequently the children interacted with nurses then the more they trusted nurses. Broadly, the findings support the conclusion that children's trust in health professionals (physicians and nurses) promotes physical health.

DOES A PERSON'S TRUST IN HIS OR HER MARRIAGE PARTNER PROMOTE HIS OR HER HEALTH?

An answer to this question is provided in the study by Schneider, Konijn, Righetti, and Rusbult (2011). At 26 years of age, individuals from married couples were administered the Faith-Romance Trust Scale (Rempel et al., 1985, see Chapter 5), a physical health scale (33 potential health problems), and evaluations of measures of mental health (depression and anxiety). The couples were administered these across five successive 6-month time periods. It was found that trust in a romantic partner longitudinally predicted self-reported health and the findings supported the conclusion that trust in marriage partners is a probable cause of health. Furthermore, the findings showed that that relation was mediated by mental health (low anxiety and depression), which supported the conclusion that trust caused health, in part, because it promoted mental health.

WHAT ROLE DOES TRUST PLAY IN EATING DISORDERS?

Obesity is regarded as an epidemic in the United Kingdom and the United States, as well as around the world (Hruby & Hu, 2015). Less prevalent but still a serious problem are the eating disorders of anorexia nervosa, bulimia nervosa, and binge eating disorders. Anorexia nervosa is diagnosed, in part, from a body mass index of less than 85% and severe and selective restriction of food intake. Bulimia nervosa is diagnosed, in part, as attempts to restrict food intake that are punctuated by repeated binges and self-induced vomiting. By the age of 20, 15% of women have one of these three eating disorders (Stice, Marti, & Rohde, 2013). The percentage is about half of that for men.

All types of eating disorders pose risks to mental and physical health. Obesity increases the risk of heart disease and diabetes (Yan et al., 2004) and psychological problems such as depression (Papadopoulos & Brennan, 2015). Studies show that those with anorexia nervosa, bulimia nervosa, and binge eating disorders are inclined to have psychological problems (e.g., depression, loneliness), and suicidal tendencies (Fairburn & Harrison, 2003).

My colleagues and I have examined the role of trust in eating disorders and health as part of the Social Withdrawal Syndrome (SWS). The SWS comprises a coherent pattern of low trust beliefs in others, low disclosure to others, and heightened loneliness. In one study, we found that bulimic symptoms in young adults were associated with low trust beliefs in close others (mother, father, and friends), an unwillingness to disclose personal information to them, and high loneliness (Rotenberg et al., 2013). In a re-analysis of that data using Body Mass Index (BMI), we found that obese individuals similarly showed the SWS pattern (Rotenberg, Bharathi, Davies, & Finch, 2017). In another study, my colleagues and I found that low trust beliefs in close others (mother, father, and friend) by early adolescents (11 to 12 years of age) predicted an increase in their bulimic symptoms across a 5-month period (Rotenberg & Sangha, 2015). Also, we found that that predictive relation was due, in part, to the relation between low trust beliefs and loneliness. Overall, the findings support the hypothesis that bulimia nervosa and obesity are associated with the Social Withdrawal Syndrome. Also, we proposed that because of the SWS, those with eating disorders were at risk for psychological and physical health problems, The SWS caused them to withhold information about their eating and emotional problems from health professionals which decreased the likelihood that they would be treated for their problems.

ARE THERE CONSEQUENCES OF BEING TOO TRUSTING IN THE MEDICAL PROFESSION?

It may be posed that being highly trusting in medical professionals makes an individual too passive, too gullible, and unengaged in interactions with health professionals – all of which would decrease the likelihood of proper medical treatment. This view is frequently raised by authors who advocate that medical/health education and information be provided to patients in order to empower them and increase their chances of receiving proper medical treatment (see Pilgrim, Tomasini, & Vassilev, 2010). As yet, researchers have not reported curvilinear relationships between trust beliefs in health professionals and health behaviours. One promising approach to this issue resides in the implementation of a physician-patient working alliance that entails empathy, trust, and shared decision-making in physician-patient relationships. The physician-patient working alliance has been found to be associated with patient adherence, satisfaction, and improved patient outcomes (see Fuertes, Toporovsky, Reyes, & Osborne, 2017). These findings may be interpreted as indicating that some blend of patients' trust in physicians and shared decision-making with physicians is optimally associated with health.

SUMMARY

This chapter reviews the research showing that generalised trust, trust in health professionals, and trust in romantic partners are associated with health (e.g., longevity and adherence to prescribed medical regimes). The chapter addressed the apparent racial disparities of HIV treatment and trust in physicians, as well as the relation between eating disorders and the lack of trust. The chapter culminates in describing physician-patient working alliance programs as an important blend of trust and joint decision-making in medical treatment.

REFERENCES

Barefoot, J. C., Maynard, K. E., Beckham, J. C., Brammett, B. H., Hooker, K., & Siegler, I. C. (1998). Trust, health and longevity. *Journal of Behavioral Medicine*, 21, 517–526.

Birkhäuer, J., Gaab, J., Kossowsky, J., Hasler, S., Krummenacher, P., Werner, C., & Gerger, H. (2017). Trust in the health care professional and health outcome: A meta-analysis. *PLoS ONE*, 12(2), 1–13. doi:10.1371/journal.pone.0170988

Blendon, R. J., Benson, J. M., & Hero, J. O. (2014). Public trust in physicians – U.S. medicine in international perspective. *New England Journal of Medicine*, 371, 1570–1572. doi:10.1056/NEJMp1407373

Fairburn, C. G., & Harrison, P. J. (2003). Eating disorders. *Lancet*, 361(9355), 407–417.

Fuertes, J. N., Toporovsky, A., Reyes, M., & Osborne, J. B. (2017, April). The physician-patient working alliance: Theory, research, and future possibilities. *Patient Education and Counseling*, 100(4), 610–615. doi:10.1016/j.pec.2016.10.018

Harding, A. (2014, October). *American's trust in doctors is failing*. Retrieved from www.livescience.com/48407-americans-trust-doctors-falling.html

Hruby, A., & Hu, F. (2015). The epidemiology of obesity: A big picture *Pharmaco Economics*, 33(7), 673–689. doi:10.1007/s40273–014–0243-x

Nummela, O., Raivio, R., & Uutela, A. (2012). Trust, self-rated health and mortality: A longitudinal study among ageing people in Southern Finland. *Social Science & Medicine*, 74(10), 1639–1643. doi http://dx.doi.org/10.1016/j.socscimed.2012.02.010

Papadopoulos, S., & Brennan, L. (2015). Correlates of weight stigma in adults with overweight and obesity: A systematic literature review. *Obesity*, 23(9), 1743–1760. doi:http://dx.doi.org/10.1002/oby.21187

Pilgrim, D., Tomasini, F., & Vassilev, I. (2010). *Examining trust in healthcare: A multidisciplinary perspective*. London: Palgrave Macmillan.

Rempel, J. K., Holmes, J. G., & Zanna, M. P. (1985). Trust in close relationships. *Journal of Personality and Social Psychology*, 49(1), 95–112.

Rotenberg, K. J., Bharathi, C., Davies, H., & Finch, T. (2013). Bulimic symptoms and the social withdrawal syndrome. *Eating Behaviors*, 14(3), 281–284. doi:http://dx.doi.org/10.1016/j.eatbeh.2013.05.003

Rotenberg, K. J., Bharathi, C., Davies, H., & Finch, T. (2017). Obesity and the social withdrawal syndrome. *Eating Behaviors*, 26, 167–170. doi: org/10.1016/j.eatbeh.2017.03.006

Rotenberg, K. J., Cunningham, J., Hayton, N., Hutson, L., Jones, L., Marks, C. Woods, E., & Betts, L. R. (2008). Development of a children's trust in general physicians scale. *Child: Health, Care and Development*, 34, 748–756. doi:10.1111/j.1365-2214.2008.00872.x

Rotenberg, K. J., & Sangha, R. (2015). Bulimic symptoms and social withdrawal during early adolescence. *Eating Behaviors*, 19, 177–180. doi:http://dx.doi.org/10.1016/j.eatbeh.2015.09.008

Rotenberg, K. J., Woods, E., & Betts, L. R. (2015). Development of a scale to assess children's trust in general nurses. *Journal of Specialists in Pediatric Nursing*, 20(4), 298–303. doi:10.1111/jspn.12126

Saha, S., Jacobs, E. A., Moore, R. D., & Beach, M. C. (2010). Trust in physicians and racial disparities in HIV care. *AIDS Patient Care and STDs*, 24(7), 415–420. doi:10.1089/apc.2009.0288

Schneider, I. K., Konijn, E. A., Righetti, F., & Rusbult, C. E. (2011). A healthy dose of trust: The relationship between interpersonal trust and health. *Personal Relationships*, 18(4), 668–676. doi:10.1111/j.1475-6811.2010.01338.x

Stice, E., Marti, N., & Rohde, P. (2013). Prevalence, incidence, impairment, and course of the proposed DSM-5 eating disorder diagnoses in an 8-year prospective community study of young women. *Journal of Abnormal Psychology*, 122(2), 445–457. doi:http://dx.doi.org/10.1037/a0030679

Thom, D. H., Kravitz, R. L., Bell, R. A., Krupat, E., & Azari, R. (2002). Patient trust in the physician: Relationship to patient requests. *Family Practice*, 19(5), 476–483.

Thom, D. H., Ribisl, K. M., Stewart, A. L., Luke, D. A., & The Stanford Trust Study Physicians. (1999). Further validation and reliability testing of the trust in physician scale. *Medical Care*, 37(5), 510–517.

Yan, L. L., Daviglus, M. L., Liu, K., Pirzada, A., Garside, D. B., Schiffer, L., Dyer, A. R., & Greenland, P. (2004). BMI and health-related quality of life in adults 65 years and older. *Obesity Research*, 12(1), 69–76.